IBN AL-JAZZĀR ON FEVERS

This volume is part of a highly important work—*Zād al-musāfir wa-qūt al-ḥāḍir*—compiled by the Arab physician Ibn al-Jazzār of Qayrawān in the tenth century. Consisting of seven books that provide concise descriptions and discussions of different diseases and their treatment, from head to toe, it was one of the most influential medical handbooks in medieval Europe. Ibn al-Jazzār's *Zād al-musāfir* not only offered a traditional pathology, but also introduced new objects of reflection, such as mental pathology, to the Western physician for the first time. It contains many valuable quotations from the works of ancient and medieval physicians and philosophers such as Aristotle, Rufus, Galen, Polemon, Paul of Aegina and Qusṭā ibn Lūqā which, in several cases, are only preserved in this work.

The section from *Zād al-musāfir* presented here is the seventh book, consisting of six chapters dealing with all the different simple kinds of fever known in his time. It is the first time one of the medical works of the Arab physicians dealing with fevers has been published in a critical edition and translation. This important work represents a great advance in the understanding of Islamic and Western medicine.

THE AUTHOR

Gerrit Bos is an expert on the history of medieval medicine, particularly as found in Hebrew and Arabic texts. He is the author of *Ibn al-Jazzār on Forgetfulness and its Treatment*, *Ibn al-Jazzār on Sexual Diseases and their Treatment* and, with Charles Burnett, of a work on medieval weather forecasting, with reference to the work of al-Kindī. Gerrit Bos has a PhD from the Vrije Universiteit in Amsterdam and currently holds the chair in Jewish Studies at the Martin Buber Institute, University of Cologne, Germany.

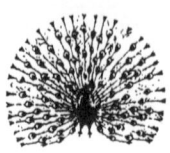

THE SIR HENRY WELLCOME
ASIAN SERIES

IBN AL-JAZZĀR ON FEVERS

A critical edition of *Zād al-musāfir wa-qūt al-ḥāḍir*

Provisions for the Traveller and Nourishment for the sedentary
Book 7, Chapters 1-6

The original Arabic text
With an English translation, introduction and commentary
by
GERRIT BOS

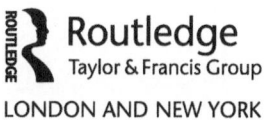

Routledge
Taylor & Francis Group

LONDON AND NEW YORK

First published in 2000 by
Kegan Paul International

2 Park Square, Milton Park, Abingdon, Oxon OX14 4RN
711 Third Avenue, New York, NY 10017, USA

Routledge is an imprint of the Taylor & Francis Group, an informa business

First issued in paperback 2016

Copyright © Gerrit Bos 2000

British Library Cataloguing in Publication Data
A catalogue record for this book is available from the British Library

ISBN 978-1-138-97218-6 (pbk)
ISBN 978-0-7103-0570-1 (hbk)

Publisher's Note
The publisher has gone to great lengths to ensure the quality of this reprint
but points out that some imperfections in the original copies may be
apparent. The publisher has made every effort to contact original copyright
holders and would welcome correspondence from those they have been
unable to trace.

PREFACE

As part of my ongoing interest in Ibn al-Jazzār's medical compendium, called *Zād al-musāfir wa-qūt al-ḥāḍir (Provisions for the Traveller and Nourishment for the Sedentary)* I would like to present to the reader a critical edition with translation and introduction of the section from Bk. 7, chs. 1-6 which deals with the different kinds of fevers. Such an edition is an urgent desideratum in the history of Islamic medicine, since so far none of the medical works of the Islamic physicians dealing with fevers has been published in a critical edition and translation.

Ibn al-Jazzār's *Zād al-musāfir* is one of the most influential medical handbooks in the history of Western medicine. Already in the beginning of the 11th century it was translated into Greek. In the 12th century Constantine the African translated it into Latin; this translation was the basis for the commentaries of the Salernitan masters from the 13th century on. As part of the so-called *Articella* or *Ars medicinae*, a compendium of medical textbooks, it was widely consulted in medical schools (Salerno, Montpellier), and in universities (Bologna, Paris, Oxford). It was popular in Jewish circles as well, as is attested by the fact that it was translated three times into Hebrew.

At this occasion I thank the Trust of The Wellcome Foundation for giving me the opportunity to prepare this edition by means of a Research Fellowship at the Wellcome Institute for the History of Medicine. I thank Dr Charles Burnett for reviewing the English section of the manuscript.

CONTENTS

Preface   v

Introduction

   1. Biography   1

   2. MSS consulted for the edition   2

   3. Survey and evaluation of the contents of book seven,
   chs. 1-6 of *Zād al-musāfir*   5

Arabic text   23

Translation   97

Glossary of materia medica   139

Glossary of technical terms (Arabic)   151

Index of proper names (Arabic)   193

Glossary of technical terms (English)   195

Index of proper names (English)   211

Bibliography   213

INTRODUCTION

1. *Biography*

Abū Jaʿfar Aḥmad b. Abī Khālid ibn al-Jazzār (10th century), a
practising physician from Qayrawān, the medieval capital of
Tunisia was a prolific author in the field of medicine. His most
famous work is beyond any doubt *Zād al-musāfir wa-qūt al-ḥāḍir*
(Provisions for the Traveller and Nourishment for the
Sedentary), a medical compendium in seven books dealing with
all the diseases *a capite ad calcem* (from head to toe).[1] This
work is for the major part still in manuscript; only books one to
three have so far been edited by Suwaysī-al-Rādī.[2] A critical
edition and translation of book six dealing with sexual diseases
has been prepared by the present author. The section on fevers
covers chs. 1-6 of book seven of Ibn al-Jazzār's *Zād al-musāfir*.
I have decided to edit this section on its own since it is an
independent unit dealing with all the different (simple) fevers
known in his days.[3] Such an edition is a desideratum, since so
far none of the medical works of the Islamic physicians dealing
with fevers has been published in a critical edition and

---

[1] For his biographical and bibliographical data see my *Ibn al-Jazzār on
women's diseases and their treatment*, pp. 296-297, and especially the
introduction to my edition and translation of book six of *Zād al-musāfir*.

[2] Ed. Tunis 1986. For a critical evaluation of this edition see my edition
of book six.

[3] He omitted the mixed fevers probably in conformity with his aim to
compose a concise practical handbook.

translation.[4]

2. *MSS consulted for the edition*

The present edition is based on the following manuscripts:

1. Berlin 252 (=Qu 683); Judaeo-Arabic. Bk. 7, chs. 1-6 cover fols.130-144; the text is written in a clear oriental script. It was probably copied in the 14th-15th cent. In my edition it bears the sign B.[5]

2. Dresden 209; the *Zād* covers 303 folios. Bk. 7, chs. 1-6 cover fols. 248-267; this manuscript is in general not very correct; it is unvocalised, while diacritical points are sometimes omitted and often confused. It has been copied by four different hands: a. from fols. 1-78, the handwriting is rather correct; b. fols. 79-269, different handwriting, very untidy in fols. 250-260; c. fols. 270-288, different handwriting, regular and correct; d. fols. 290-339, different rather careless handwriting; fols. 290 and 291 contain marginal passages taken from the Koran as a remedy for scabies, probably added by a pious copyist; the copying of the manuscript was completed in the year 1091/1680. In my text edition it is indicated by the sign D.[6]

---

[4] The only partial edition I know about is that by Latham-Isaacs which deals with the section on "sill" (consumption) from *K. al-ḥummāyāt* by Isḥāq ibn Sulaymān al-Isrā'īlī.

[5] See Steinschneider, *Die hebräischen Handschriften in Berlin*, 104, no. 252; idem, *Schriften der Araber in hebräischen Handschriften*, 346; Ullmann, *Die Medizin im Islam*, p. 147, n. 6.

[6] See Fleischer, *Catalogus codicum manuscriptorum orientalium in Bibliothecae Regiae Dresdensis*, 31-2; Dugat, *Études*, 293-4; according to

3. Oxford, Bodleian Huntington 302. Bk. 7, chs. 1-6 cover fols. 179-195. The text, vocalised and provided with diacritical points, was copied in the year 738/1337, and is therefore the oldest surviving manuscript. It is indicated in my edition with the sign O.[7]

4. Teheran, Malik 4486; unnumbered. The text is unvocalised, but provided with diacritical points; it was copied in the year 994/1586. The copyist was rather careless and did not understand the text in hand very well; this has resulted in many corruptions and omissions. It is indicated in my edition with the sign T.[8]

5. Izmir, Millī 50/470 (26636). Bk. 7, chs. 1-7 cover fols. 145-156. The text is partly vocalised and was copied by Zayn al-'ābidīn on 4. Shawwāl 972 H (1564).[9] In general this text provides good readings with the occasional mistake typical for a copyist. In many cases it has readings similar to those of MS Teheran, indicating a common ancestor.

I did not consult MS Copenhagen 109 and Paris 2884, since both MSS have been copied from MS Dresden.[10] MS Wellcome A 463, part of the former Sāmī Ibrahīm Ḥaddād collection and

---

Dugat (*op. cit.*, 293) the copying of this MS was completed in the year 1009/1600.

[7] See Uri, *Bibliothecae Bodleianae codicum manuscriptorum orientalium ...catalogus*, vol. 1, 133, no. 559.

[8] Cf. Sezgin, *GAS* III, 305. I thank Professor Mohaghegh for providing me with a photostat of this MS.

[9] See Dietrich, *Medicinalia Arabica*, 63-4. I thank Professor Sezgin for providing me with a photostat of book seven of this manuscript.

[10] For an extensive comparison of MSS Copenhagen and Dresden see my edition of bk. 6 of the *Zād*. For MS Paris see Vajda, *Index général des manuscrits arabes musulmans*, p. 729. Sezgin, *op. cit.*, p. 305, refers to the fact that MS Paris is a copy of Dresden.

consisting of 30 fols., only covers Bk. 1, chs. 1-18.[11] Other
MSS which I could not consult, since, despite all my efforts, I
could not obtain photostats of them, are:

1. Algiers 1746, fols. 1-75, 10 cent. H. (16th cent. A.D.).

2. Cairo VI[1], 37, *tibb*, *maj.* 37 m (fols. 1-39a, 11 cent. H.
(17th cent. A.D.).

3. Rabāt 1718 (fols. 1b-222a).[12]

My edition is mainly based on BIOT since the readings preserved
by these MSS are often better than those of MS Dresden.
Moreover, the readings preserved by these MSS represent in
many cases a more complete version than that in MS Dresden.
Unfortunately, it proved to be impossible to establish a stemma
precisely defining the relationship of these MSS, because of the
contaminated state of the tradition. The textual tradition is clearly
very complex but on the basis of the MSS available at the moment
further clarification is impossible.[13]

---

[11] Dr Conrad is preparing a catalogue describing all the MSS from this
collection acquired by the Wellcome Institute for the History of Medicine.

[12] The bibliographers mention two more MSS of the *Zād al-musāfir*, namely,
Dublin, Chester Beatty 5224, fols. 50b-88a, and Washington, Army Medical
Library 92/1, fols. 1-73. Their information, however, is incorrect. These
MSS do not contain Ibn al-Jazzār's *Zād al-musāfir* as the bibliographers
suggest, but his *Tibb al-fuqarā' wa-l-masākīn* (Medicine for the poor); see
my edition of book six for a more detailed discussion of this issue.

[13] The question of the extent to which the translations into Greek, Hebrew
and Latin could assist in this task is equally vexed. No scientific research on
the Greek tradition has been done, the Hebrew tradition consists of MSS
representing three different translations, and Constantine's Latin rendering is
a paraphrase for which, again, the state of the textual tradition is unknown.

3. *Survey and evaluation of the contents of Bk. 7, chs. 1-6 of* Zād al-musāfir

Before starting our survey one should note that Ibn al-Jazzār's major source is Galen. Like all Arabic physicians, he adopted Galen's humoral theory as the basis for his aetiology, and his therapeutical rule *contraria contrariis curantur* as the basis for the treatment of these diseases.[14] The high regard he had for Galen is clear from several quotations from his works. Moreover, in some cases, as specified in the discussion of the contents of the chapters themselves, Ibn al-Jazzār's aetiology, symptology or other specific elements are similar to those mentioned by Galen and seem to be derived from him.

In this survey I will point to sources and/or parallels from ancient and Byzantine medicine, above all Galen (2nd cent.) and Paul of Aegina (7th cent.). I will, moreover, compare Ibn al-Jazzār's discussion of the aetiology, symptology and treatment of different fevers with that of Ibn Sīnā (980-1037) and his contemporary al-Mājūsī, whose relation to Ibn al-Jazzār has not been researched so far.[15] We shall see several close parallels between these two physicians in the arrangement and contents of their subject matter, pointing, most likely, to a common source. Both physicians, however, differ greatly in so far as Ibn al-Jazzār's discussion is usually as concise as possible, omitting issues not

---

[14] For the application of this rule in the case of fevers see Galen, *Ad Glauconem de methodo medendi* I, ch. 10 (Kühn X, p. 32).

[15] See Green, *The transmission of ancient theories of female physiology and disease through the early Middle Ages*, pp. 128-129, n. 110.

relevant for a practising physician, while al-Mājūsī aims at treating
every issue, both theoretical and practical, as thorougly as possible.
In this aspect al-Mājūsī's methods and aims are similar to those
of Ibn Sīnā.

Reviewing Ibn al-Jazzār's discussion of the different fevers,
it is clear that he almost invariably adheres to a certain scheme.
First of all, he gives a very concise aetiology, then a more extensive
symptology, while most of his attention goes to the different
ways of treatment of the disease. Within this scheme he has,
moreover, organised the material in a very logical and
comprehensible way. He has thus met the aim which he set
himself for the composition of the *Zād al-musāfir*:

> I have seen how many great and excellent physicians have composed
> books on the treatment of the diseases which may affect each of the
> limbs [of the body], with the intention of composing a work fitted for
> regular consultation. Some of these works, however, are longer and more
> detailed than necessary, while others are shorter than necessary. Knowing
> this, I have composed a work on the treatment of the diseases which may
> affect each of the limbs of the body and I have called it "Zād al-musāfir
> wa-qūt al-ḥāḍir". I left out everything that might spoil it by making it too
> burdensome, too long, too complicated and too profound. Word of it
> spread in the countries and it was well received by the physicians.[16]

As noted above, it is probably precisely for this reason that Ibn
al-Jazzār chose not to discuss the mixed fevers, since their
diagnosis and treatment is too complicated. But in spite of the
good reputation which the *Zād al-musāfir* acquired for itself, Ibn
al-Jazzār was not blind to its limitations, and recognised at a

---

[16] Introduction to *Ṭibb al-fuqarā' wa-l-masākīn*, MS Paris 3038; I am
preparing a critical edition with English translation of this text; see my edition
of Bk. 6 of the *Zād* for a more extensive treatment of the subject.

certain moment the necessity for the composition of a new work, namely, the *Ṭibb al-fuqarā' wa-l-masākīn*.

Introduction

Ibn al-Jazzār introduces his discussion of fever by quoting Galen that it is "the most dangerous disease, the messenger of death, and the most frequent cause of the end of life." This kind of introduction is unusual in Islamic medical literature, for Islamic physicians usually start their discussion of fever with its definition. Ibn Sīnā, for instance, remarks: "Fever is a strange heat that burns in the heart and spreads from it through the mediation of the pneuma and the blood through the arteries and veins in the whole body."[17] And al-Mājūsī remarks that fever "is a disease arising from a hot dyscrasia and encompassing the whole body and that it is an unnatural heat arising from the heart and passing from the arteries and veins into all the organs of the body."[18]

These definitions go back to Galen, according to whom fever is an unnatural heat affecting the body.[19] However, the next phrases in Ibn al-Jazzār's introduction, that fever "encompasses both the external and internal [parts of] the body" and that "it is harmful for the pneumata, the psychical faculties, and the natural activities [of the body]" are similar to those of Ibn Sīnā and

---

[17] Ibn Sinā, *K. al-Qānūn fī l-ṭibb*, Bk. 4, discourse 1, ch. 1, p. 2.

[18] Al-Mājūsī, *Kāmil al-ṣinā'a al-ṭibbīya*, Bk. 1, discourse 8, ch. 2, p. 347.

[19] *De febrium differentiis*, I, ch. 2 (Kühn VII, p. 277); *Über die medizinischen Namen*, p. 19 (Arabic text p. 9); cf. Brain, *Galen on bloodletting*, p. 10. Brain rightly remarks that since in Galen's system all fevers are pathological dyscrasias of the Hot, he would not have agreed with the modern idea, which some of the ancients seem to have held also, that fever is a beneficial adaptation.

al-Mājūsī. For Ibn Sīnā remarks that fever is harmful for the natural activities (*taḍurru bi l-afʿāl al-ṭabīʿiya*), while al-Mājūsī holds that it is harmful for the activities of the organs.[20] It is clear that Ibn al-Jazzār decided not to start his discourse with a definition of fever but by quoting his revered master and the most authoritative source of Islamic physicians in general.

For it is on Galen that Ibn al-Jazzār's discussion of the different kinds of fever is based. Galen divided fevers into three kinds, namely, that due to a temporary overheating of the body, the result of some external cause, the simplest variety of which is the ephemeral, and those caused by inflammation or putrefaction of residues that have accumulated within the body.[21] A three-fold division of fevers recurs in al-Mājūsī's encyclopaedia where he distinguishes between fever occurring in the pneuma (which is called ephemeral fever), fever occurring in the humours (which is called putrefactive fever), and fever occurring in the main organs (which is called hectic fever).[22]

Ibn Sīnā refers to different divisions of fevers. One of these is a division into two kinds, namely, original and accidental fever (*ḥumā maraḍ wa-ḥumā ʿaraḍ*). Another division is one into three kinds: hectic fever (*ḥumā diqq*); humoral fever (*ḥumā ḥalaṭ*); and ephemeral fever (*ḥumā yawm*). About this division Ibn Sīnā remarks that it is closely related to the division of the seasons. In Ibn al-Jazzār's survey of the different fevers we can discern a two-fold division, distinguishing between fevers

---

[20] Ibn Sīnā, *ibid.* Al-Mājūsī, *ibid.*

[21] See Galen, *De methodo medendi* X, ch. 1 (Kühn X, pp. 661-663); Brain, *op. cit.*, p. 13; Langermann, *Maimonides on the synochous fever*, pp. 179-180.

[22] Al-Mājūsī, *ibid.*

originating from the pneumata and fevers originating from the humours (yellow bile, blood, black bile, humoral phlegm).

Chapter one

The subject of this chapter is ephemeral fever. This fever came to denote, as Latham and Isaacs remark, "'milk-fever' in modern medicine, a slight feverish attack occurring about the third or fourth day after childbirth."[23] We have seen above that al-Mājūsī also refers to the pneuma as the place of origin of this fever. About its length Ibn al-Jazzār remarks that it does not last longer than one day. According to al-Mājūsī it lasts 24 hours, but sometimes forty-eight or even seventy-two hours;[24] according to Ibn Sīnā it usually lasts one day and rarely longer than three days.[25]

Ibn al-Jazzār divides this fever into two kinds, namely, when the fever is the disease itself (original) and when it is accidental to the disease. Ibn Sīnā mentions, as we saw above, a similar division for fevers in general. Isḥāq ibn Sulaymān al-Isrā'īlī, Ibn al-Jazzār's teacher in medicine, makes a similar distinction for "fever consequent on decline."[26]

Ibn al-Jazzār mentions three possible causes for original ephemeral fever: 1. External, the heat in the summer, a hot sandstorm, severe cold, and bathing in waters which obstruct the

---

[23] Latham-Isaacs, *op. cit.*, p. 82, n. 20.

[24] al-Mājūsī, *op. cit.*, Bk. 1, discourse 8, ch. 3, p. 348.

[25] Ibn Sīnā, *op. cit.*, Bk. 4, p. 6.

[26] *K. al-ḥummāyāt*, *op. cit.*, pp. 6-7 (Arabic); p. 7 (English translation).

pores of the skin, since they contain natron, alum, and sulphur;[27]
2. Excess of bodily movement and excessive emotions; 3.
Continuous consumption of hot food. The author thus includes
physical (external) and psychic factors in his enumeration. Al-
Mājūsī mentions four external causes similar to those enumerated
by Ibn al-Jazzār, but omits psychic factors: 1. Heat [of the sun],
heat of the bathhouse; 2. Bathing in waters mixed with hot
ingredients like sulphur; 3. That which compresses the pores
such as cold water used in a clyster; 4. Taking a bath in water
containing alum.[28] Ibn Sīnā states that this fever has different
physical and psychic causes, and that it is a mistake to think that
it only occurs after exertion of body or mind.[29] He then gives a
detailed list of 23 different types of ephemeral fever which are
called according to these causes.[30] The aetiology stated by these
physicians for this disease goes back to Galen, according to
whom ephemeral fever "is due simply to overheating of the
body by the sun, anger, exertion, heat-producing foods or drinks,
or to reduction of heat loss through insufficient transpiration
when the pores of the skin are obstructed."[31]

Ibn al-Jazzār now gives a detailed enumeration of the different
symptoms of ephemeral fever according to its different causes.
A similar enumeration is given by al-Mājūsī; however the specific
symptoms mentioned by him are partly different. For instance,

---

[27] On these kinds of waters see the extensive discussion by Qusṭā ibn
Lūqā in his *Risāla fī tadbīr safar al-ḥajj*, ch. 8.

[28] *Op. cit.*, ibid.

[29] *Op. cit.*, Bk. 4, pp. 5-6; cf. p. 8.

[30] *Op. cit.*, Bk. 4, pp. 8-16. The first type, for instance is called "ḥūmā
yawm ghamīya" (ephemeral fever caused by sorrow).

[31] Brain, *op. cit.*, p. 11.

in the case of ephemeral fever caused by the burning of the sun or hot air, he mentions the following symptoms: the eyes of the patient feel hot, his head is burning, the face and the skin are dry and feel hot, the pulse is small and fast. An important difference between both is that in al-Mājūsī's symptology the pulse figures prominently, while Ibn al-Jazzār only mentions it in the case of psychic causes. Following Galen,[32] Ibn Sīnā gives much attention to the pulse, but also to the urine.[33]

As treatment for the different kinds of ephemeral fever Ibn al-Jazzār recommends a detailed regimen for each kind, based on the general principle of "contraria contrariis curantur." Important elements are bathing of the body and/or feet in different kinds of waters;[34] errhines and diet.

Chapter two

The main topic of this chapter is ardent fever. Grmek has pointed out that it is methodologically incorrect to try to identify this disease from the viewpoint of modern pathology. Only in very specific cases can we recognise its true nature. For in the texts we have this disease-name only has a general reference.[35]

---

[32] See, for instance, *Ad Glauconem de methodo medendi* I, ch. 2 (Kühn XI, p. 8).

[33] *Op. cit.*, Bk. 4, pp. 8-16.

[34] For the importance of the bathhouse (*hammām*) in Islamic culture see Grotzfeld, *Das Bad*. For the prominent role of bathing in curing all fevers see Galen, *Ad Glauconem de methodo medendi* I, ch. 3 (Kühn XI, p. 14).

[35] Grmek, *Diseases in the ancient Greek world*, pp. 289-292. In this section entitled "*The Meaning of* Kaûsos *in Hippocratic Medicine*," Grmek has dealt exhaustively with the ancient sources discussing this disease, as well as with modern interpretations.

However, for the ancient and medieval physicians it certainly was a disease and a very dangerous one. Like some Greek and Byzantine predecessors, Ibn al-Jazzār distinguishes between two clinical forms, one authentic and severe and the other false and light. As to its causes Ibn al-Jazzār remarks that the authentic one originates from pure yellow bile that has collected in the veins adjacent to the heart, while the false one is caused by yellow bile mixed with sweet moisture or sweet vapour. Ibn Sīnā distinguishes between two kinds of ardent fever according to their causes; one is called "bilious ardent fever" and the other "mucous ardent fever".[36] This distinction can, as Grmek remarks, be found with later authors who had a tendency to reduce one of the two forms of *kausos* to disturbances in bile and the other to those in phlegm.[37] It can, for instance, be found in the medical encyclopaedia composed by Alexander of Tralles (d. 605).[38] Next to the symptoms recorded by Ibn al-Jazzār, namely, continuous heat and thirst, Ibn Sīnā mentions several others and notes that in the case of bilious ardent fever the symptoms are worse than in that of mucous ardent fever. Some of these symptoms recorded by him are insomnia, perplexity, nosebleed, headache and relaxation of the bowels.[39]

Ibn al-Jazzār introduces his recommendations for the treatment of ardent fever with a lengthy quotation from Galen about three criteria to be considered by the physician for the treatment of sharp diseases in general, namely, the degree of strength of the

---

[36] *Op. cit.*, Bk. 4, p. 38.
[37] Cf. Grmek, *op. cit.*, p. 292.
[38] Ed. Puschmann, vol. 1, p. 323.
[39] *Op. cit.*, Bk. 4, p. 38.

patient to fight the disease, the duration of the disease, and the quality of the disease.[40] The amount of food should be in proportion to his strength; the quality of the food should be according to the nearness or distance of the crisis of the disease, and the general regimen should be related to the quality of the disease. Al-Mājūsī remarks on the regimen for fevers in general that it should be according to the nature of the fever, the times (phases) of the fever, the strength of the patient, the health of the body [of the patient], the appetite [of the patient], the times of the crises [of the fever]. One should also consider those factors that prevent the patient from taking food.[41]

As for ardent fever in particular, Ibn al-Jazzār remarks that since this fever is very dangerous and frightening, the physician should proceed in it very carefully from the beginning, he should observe the four phases of a disease, namely, beginning, progress, crisis and abatement, and apply in every phase that which is necessary. The concept of the four phases of a disease is discussed extensively by Galen,[42] and is common in Islamic medicine.[43]

Hereafter Ibn al-Jazzār gives detailed prescriptions for the case that the ardent fever is high and severe from the beginning, and for ardent fever accompanied by constipation, insomnia, palpitation, phrenitis, dry cough, fainting, or jaundice. Ibn Sīnā

---

[40] This quotation is not from Galen's *De crisibus* as adduced by Ibn al-Jazzār, but probably an adaptation of Galen's commentary on Hippocrates' *De victu acutorum*, ed. Helmreich II 36, 580, pp. 194-195. I thank Professor Vivian Nutton for this reference.

[41] *Op. cit.*, Bk. 2, discourse 3, ch. 11, p. 229.

[42] *De totius morbi temporibus* (Kühn VII, pp. 440-462); *De crisibus* I, ch. 2 (Kühn IX; pp. 551-552); cf. Paul of Aegina, Bk. 2, ch. 4.

[43] Cf. Ibn Sīnā, *op. cit.*, Bk. 1, p. 78.

first of all recommends treating the patient in the same way as in the case of pure tertian fever and then proceeds with detailed prescriptions; like Ibn al-Jazzār he gives different prescriptions for different symptoms.[44]

Chapter 3

In this chapter Ibn al-Jazzār discusses tertian fever. Its cause is, according to him, putrefied yellow bile. Paul of Aegina and al-Mājūsī refer to a similar cause.[45] Ibn al-Jazzār's distinction between putrefaction outside the veins and arteries and causing intermittent tertian fever, and putrefaction inside the veins and arteries, causing either continuous tertian fever or burning fever, has a close parallel in al-Mājūsī.[46]

Symptoms enumerated by Ibn al-Jazzār are cold, shuddering and tremor, vomiting, diarrhoea, red fiery and fine urine, intense blazing heat and a pricking sensation in the liver. Some of these symptoms are mentioned by Galen[47] and Paul of Aegina,[48] while Ibn Sīnā adds many others and especially stresses the changes in the condition of the pulse.[49] Ibn al-Jazzār mentions three

---

[44] *Op. cit.*, Bk. 4, pp. 38-39.

[45] Paul of Aegina, *De re medica*, Bk. 2, ch. 18, speaks of "moving yellow bile", and al-Mājūsī refers to putrefied yellow bile (*Op. cit.*, Bk. 1, discourse 8, ch. 4, p. 351).

[46] *Op. cit.*, Bk. 1, discourse 8, ch. 4, p. 352. Al-Mājūsī says that this distinction holds good for all fevers originating from the putrefaction of one of the humours. Galen distinguished between intermittent tertian fever and continous semi tertian fever; see *Über die medizinischen Namen*, p. 10, n. 5.

[47] *De crisibus* II, ch. 3, (Kühn IX, pp. 656-657).

[48] *Op. cit.*, Bk. 2, ch. 18.

[49] *Op. cit*, Bk. 4, p. 34.

kinds of things indicating tertian fever: 1. Natural: the patient has a hot and dry temperament, is between twenty and thirty-five years old and his body is lean with open pores; 2. Unnatural: hot and dry weather (summer), the patient has a hard profession; 3. Extra-natural: the symptoms mentioned above. The distinction between natural and unnatural indications also occurs in al-Mājūsī's encyclopaedia .[50]

Ibn al-Jazzār's classification is based on Galen, according to whom tertian fever only occurs to a patient whose body is of a bilious nature, and who is in the prime of his life. It occurs, he says, especially during the summer in hot and dry countries with hot and dry weather to a patient whose mode of life is not in idleness but in hardship, anxiety, insomnia, sunburn, and little food that is hot and dry.[51]

Ibn al-Jazzār distinguishes between two types of tertian fever, pure and impure. The pure type mostly lasts for twelve hours and its abatement lasts for thirty-six hours; its maximum number of bouts is seven. The impure type lasts longer and has more than seven bouts. Galen,[52] Paul of Aegina[53] and Ibn Sīnā[54] use similar criteria for distinguishing between pure and impure tertian fever. Ibn al-Jazzār also remarks that if the tertian is impure and

---

[50] *Op. cit.*, Bk. 1, discourse 8, ch. 5, p. 354.

[51] *De febrium differentiis* II, ch. 1 (Kühn VII, p. 334); cf. *De crisibus* II, ch. 3 (Kühn IX, p. 657); *Ad Glauconem de methodo medendi* I, ch. 5 (Kühn XI, pp. 19-20).

[52] *De febrium differentiis* II, ch. 3 (Kühn VII, p. 339); cf. *Ad Glauconem de methodo medendi* I, ch. 9 (Kühn XI, p. 29). In *Über die medizinischen Namen*, p. 10 (Arabic text p. 3), Galen refers to a tertian fever lasting for twenty-six hours and abating for twenty-two hours.

[53] *Op. cit.*, Bk. 2, ch. 18.

[54] *Op. cit,* Bk. 4, pp. 34-35.

combined with another fever, it exceeds the limit of the impure
type and will last even longer; sometimes it will start in the
autumn and only abate in the [next] spring.

For the treatment of tertian fever and especially to extinguish
the heat and extract the sickening fluid, Ibn al-Jazzār gives, like
Ibn Sīnā[55] and al-Mājūsī,[56] lengthy detailed prescriptions
consisting of cooling drinks, decoctions, purgations, suppositories, clysters, foot-baths and diet. A similar treatment is
recommended by Galen in his *Ad Glauconem de methodo
medendi*.[57]

Chapter 4

The main subject of this chapter is blood fever (synochous
fever) caused by putrefaction of the blood within the veins and
arteries. Ibn al-Jazzār introduces his discussion of this disease
with a statement about the role and importance of blood for the
functioning of the body. It is the substance with which the body
feeds itself and by which it subsists, since it is the best balanced
element, sweetest in taste. This concept goes back to Galen[58]
and became dominant in Islamic medicine.[59] Galen's view about
the quality of blood as intrinsically well-tempered contrary to

---

[55] *Op. cit.*, Bk. 4, pp. 35-38.

[56] *Op. cit.*, Bk. 2, discourse 2, chs. 12-13; pp. 234-241.

[57] *Ad Glauconem de methodo medendi* I, chs. 10-11, (Kühn XI, pp. 32-37.)

[58] *Hippocratis de natura hominis liber primus et Galeni in eum commentarius* (Kühn XV, p. 88; Mewaldt I 37, pp. 46-47); cf. *De temperamentis* (Kühn I, pp. 524-535); Brain, *op. cit*, pp. 7-8 and Langermann, *Maimonides on the synochous fever*, pp. 180-181 treat this subject extensively.

[59] See Ullmann, *Islamic medicine*, pp. 58-59; 64-65.

the three other humours which are ill-tempered and thus can give rise to different diseases when they are excessive, points to an inconsistency in his system. For if blood is intrinsically well-tempered, how can an abundance of blood lead to a disease, as Galen thought? This inconsistency was already observed by Ibn al-Jazzār's teacher Ishāq ibn Sulaymān al-Isrā'īlī.[60] Following his teacher, Ibn al-Jazzār solves this problem by stating that when blood becomes too plentiful, nature stops regulating it, so that it deteriorates and putrefies. Nature is like a father who is forced to dislike and turn away from his favourite son because of his disobedience.[61]

As a quotation by Ibn al-Jazzār from Galen's *De febrium differentiis* shows clearly, the latter did not restrict the term synochous fever to blood fever only, but used it for all putrefying fevers originating within the arteries and veins.[62] However, in his *Ad Glauconem de methodo medendi* Galen differentiates between synochous fever resulting from a blockage of the pores of the body without putrefaction of the humours which belongs to the genus of ephemeral fevers and synochous fever originating from a blockage with putrefaction which belongs to the genus of putrefying fevers.[63] Alexander of Tralles distinguishes between blood fever caused by putrefied blood and that caused by yellow

---

[60] See Langermann, *op. cit.*, pp. 180-181.

[61] *Ibid.*

[62] *De febrium differentiis* II, ch. 1 (Kühn VII, pp. 335-336). Langermann, *op. cit.*, p. 181 suggests that restriction to blood fever only happened in late antiquity. See as well idem, pp. 186-188 for a summary of Maimonides' criticism of Galen's discussion of putrefying fevers.

[63] *De methodo medendi* IX (Kühn X, pp. 604-605); see Langermann, *op. cit.*, p. 185; cf. Paul of Aegina, *op. cit.*, Bk. 2, ch. 27.

bile.[64] Ibn al-Jazzār differentiates between blood fever originating from the putrefaction of the blood and blood fever not originating from the putrefaction of the blood but from its boiling, and mostly followed by asthma. Ancient physicians, he says, called this fever "asthmatic heat". Ibn Sīnā makes a similar distinction.[65] Al-Mājūsī remarks that synochous fever is caused by putrefied blood and that it is dangerous because it does not abate.[66]

Ibn al-Jazzār mentions two kinds of symptoms for blood fever, namely, those preceding the actual occurrence of the disease, such as indolence, heaviness and fullness of the body, a red colour and heat, and symptoms following its occurrence, such as headache, inflammation, a fast powerful pulse, red urine. Ibn Sīnā[67] and al-Mājūsī[68] mention similar symptoms without this kind of differentiation. For its treatment Ibn al-Jazzār recommends first of all bleeding or venesection for the extraction of the superfluous blood when the strength of the patient, his age, temperament, and the time of the year are favourable. Al-Mājūsī introduces his discussion of the treatment of this fever in a similar way.[69] Ibn Sīnā remarks the patient should be bled until he faints.[70] Other means recommended by Ibn al-Jazzār are cooling drinks, fine foodstuff, suppositories and clysters.[71]

---

[64] *Op. cit.*, vol. 1, p. 325.

[65] *Op. cit.*, Bk. 4, pp. 39-40.

[66] Op. cit., Bk. 1, discourse 8, ch. 4, p. 351.

[67] *Op. cit.*, Bk. 4, pp. 40-41.

[68] *Op. cit.*, Bk. 1, discourse 8, ch. 5, p. 356.

[69] *Op. cit.*, Bk. 2, discourse 3, ch. 16, p. 248.

[70] *Op. cit.*, Bk. 4, pp. 41. Paul of Aegina (*op. cit.*, Bk. 2, ch. 27) gives exactly the same advice.

[71] For Ibn Sīnā's treatment see *op. cit.*, Bk. 4, pp. 41-42; for al-Mājūsī see *op. cit.*, Bk. 2, discourse 3, ch. 16, pp. 248-252.

Chapter 5

The central subject of this chapter is quartan fever. Ibn al-Jazzār remarks that it is caused by the putrefaction of black bile. A similar aetiology can be found in Galen's *De febrium differentiis*[72] and is repeated by al-Mājūsī[73] and Ibn Sīnā.[74] Ibn al-Jazzār explains its name from the fact that it attacks once in every four days for twenty-four hours and abates for forty-eight hours. A similar explanation is given by al-Mājūsī.[75]

Its symptoms are, according to Ibn al-Jazzār, as in the case of tertian fever, of three kinds, namely, natural, unnatural and extra-natural. The natural symptoms relate to the condition of the patient, the unnatural to the weather, and the extra-natural to the afflictions occurring to the patient during the bout of this fever. Al-Mājūsī makes the same differentiation between natural, unnatural, and extra-natural symptoms, but arranges these in a different way. For he classifies the condition of the patient and the weather as natural and the previous regimen of the patient consisting of too much food and thus causing superfluous black bile, as unnatural. The extra-natural symptoms are subdivided by him into those preceding the actual quartan fever, namely, other fevers, and symptoms simultaneous with the quartan fever, such as pain, heaviness, severe cold, and a slow and very irregular

---

[72] *De febrium differentiis* II, chs. 1-2 (Kühn VII, pp. 335-336).
[73] *Op. cit.*, Bk. 1, discourse 8, ch. 4, p. 351.
[74] *Op. cit.*, Bk. 4, p. 51.
[75] *Op. cit.*, Bk. 1, discourse 8, ch. 4, p. 351.

pulse in the beginning of the fever.[76]

This classification is, as in the case of tertian fever, based on Galen. Having stressed the importance of the pulse for the diagnosis of this fever, he mentions other symptoms such as weather, season of the year, previous regimen of the patient, temperament of the patient, and preceding other fevers.[77] Ibn Sīnā does mention some similar symptoms, but the structure and arrangement of the material is totally different.[78]

Introducing his discussion of the treatment of this fever Ibn al-Jazzār recommends a variety of means depending on the symptoms. Some of these means are vomiting for the evacuation of the superfluous black bile, hot drinks when the patient has a cold temperament, cooling drinks when the quartan fever is preceded by tertian fever, cooling drinks and bleeding in the case that blood fever preceded the quartan fever, and laxatives or clysters in case of constipation. It is clear that the diagnosis of the particular fever preceding the actual quartan fever is of crucial importance for the correct treatment of the patient. Al-Mājūsī takes a different approach. According to him, the particular time of the year when the fever occurs is important for determining the correct treatment, next to other factors such as pulse, urine, and age of the patient.

---

[76] *Op. cit.*, Bk. 1, discourse 8, ch. 5, pp. 354-355.

[77] *De crisibus* II, ch. 4 (Kühn IX, pp. 638-639); cf. *Ad Glauconem de methodo medendi* I, ch. 6, (Kühn XI, pp. 20-21). Paul of Aegina also stresses the importance of the pulse (*op. cit.*, Bk. 2, ch. 21).

[78] *Op. cit.*, Bk. 4, pp. 52-53.

Chapter 6

In this chapter Ibn al-Jazzār discusses quotidian fever. It is caused, he says, by the putrefaction of the humoral phlegm. Galen refers to the same cause in his *De febrium differentiis*.[79] According to Ibn Sīnā it is caused by vitreous or acid phlegm.[80] Al-Mājūsī remarks that this fever is caused by putrefaction of the phlegm and calls it "the persistent one" (*al-muwāẓaba*).[81] As in the case of tertian fever, Ibn al-Jazzār distinguishes between putrefaction originating inside the arteries and veins causing quotidian fever, and putrefaction outside the arteries and veins causing intermittent fever. Al-Mājūsī applies, as we saw above, this distinction to all humoral fevers.

As in the case of tertian and quartan fever Ibn al-Jazzār distinguishes between natural, unnatural and extra-natural symptoms indicating quotidian fever. Natural symptoms are the temperament of the patient, namely, cold and moist, and his age, either young or old. Unnatural symptoms are the season of the year, namely, winter, the actual weather, cold and moist, the temperament of the country, and the way of life of the patient, namely, one of comfort and rest. Extra-natural symptoms are the afflictions occurring to the patient during the bout of this fever. Al-Mājūsī makes the same classification, but considers, as in the case of quartan fever, weather conditions as natural, regimen of

---

[79] *De febrium differentiis* II, ch. 1 (Kühn VII, p. 335).
[80] *Op. cit.*, Bk. 4, p. 42.
[81] *Op. cit.*, Bk. 1, discourse 8, ch. 4, p. 351.

the patient as unnatural, and the afflictions occurring to him as extra-natural.[82] This classification is based on Galen who enumerates similar symptoms in *De febrium differentiis*.[83]

As with the other putrifying fevers, the treatment of quotidian fever recommended by Ibn al-Jazzār consists foremost of different means such as emetics, decoctions, and purgatives in order to extinguish its heat and extract the superfluous phlegm. This goal is explicitly mentioned by al-Mājūsī in the introduction to his recommendations for the treatment of this fever.[84] To achieve the same goal Galen recommends administering to the patient oxymel to extinguish the heat and other drugs to expel the phlegm.[85]

---

[82] *Ibid.*, p. 355.

[83] *De febrium differentiis* II, ch. 1 (Kühn VII, pp. 334-335); cf. *Ad Glauconem de methodo medendi* I, ch. 7, (Kühn XI, pp. 22-24).

[84] *Op. cit.*, Bk. 2, discourse 3, ch. 15, pp. 245-247.

[85] *Ad Glauconem de methodo medendi* I, ch. 13 (Kühn XI, pp. 22-24).

ARABIC TEXT

Sigla and abbreviations:

B	= Berlin 252 (14th-15th cent.)
B¹	= Note in the margin of B
D	= Dresden 209 (1091/1680)
D¹	= Note in the margin of D
I	= Izmir, Milli 50/470 (972/1564)
I¹	= Note in the margin of I
O	= Oxford, Bodleian Huntington 302 (738/1337)
O¹	= Note in the margin of O
T	= Teheran, Malik 4486 (994/1586)
T¹	= Note in the margin of T
<>	= addendum
+	= addidit
-	= omisit
*	= conieci vel correxi
inv.	= invertit
ditt.	= dittography
(!)	= corrupt reading
(?)	= doubtful reading

بسم اللّه الرحمن الرحيم

المقالة[1] السابعة[2] من[3] كتاب زاد المسافر[4]

قـد أتينا بحمـد اللّه وعـونه[5] في المقالات المتقدّمـة من هذا
الكتاب على ذكر الأدواء التي[6] تعرض في الأعضاء الباطنة
وشـرحنا[7] مـداوات[8] تلك الأدواء على أهدى[9] سبله وأقـصد
طرقـه[10] وأقـرب مـأخـذه.[11] وأنا الآن ذاكـر في هذه المقالة
السابعة التي جعلتها[12] خاتمة هذا الكتاب الشريف الأدواء
الظاهرة التي تدرك بالحسّ والأدواء[13] الظاهرة التي تشـرك[14]

---

[1] المقالة: ابتداء المقالة I

[2] السابعة + وهي خاتمة الكتاب الذي ألّفه أحمد بن إبراهيم بن أبي خالد بن
الجزار في علاج اللاذواء التي تعرض في جميع أعضـاء البدن قال أحمد بن
إبراهيم T + وهي خاتمة الكتاب D

[3] من كتاب زاد المسافر: فنقول I

[4] المسافر + قال أبو جعفر أحمد ابن إبراهيم مؤلّف هذا الكتاب B

[5] وعونه: ونعمته DIT

[6] التي....الأدواء: -OT

[7] وشرحنا + طريق DI

[8] مداوات تلك الأدواء: مداواتها I

[9] أهدى سبله: أهون سبيلة D

[10] طرقه: طريقة B

[11] مأخذه: مأخذ I

[12] جعلتها: جعلناها DOT

[13] والأدواء: بالأعضاءB

بألمها[1] الأعضاء الباطنة وطريق مداواتها على المنهج الطبّي والقانون الصناعي.

ونبتدئ بذكر الحمّى فإنّها فيما ذكر جالينوس أعظم الأمراض خطرا وهي بريد[2] الموت وأكثر أسباب الأجل وذلك لأنّها[3] تشتمل باطن[4] الجسد وظاهره وتضرّ بالأرواح والقوّى[5] النفسانية والأفعال الطبيعية. ونجعل ابتداء كلامنا في حمّى يوم المتولّدة في الأرواح[6] وذلك لأنّ[7] هذه الحمّى كثيرا ما تعرض من أدنى سبب وهي كثيرا ما تكون سببا لحدوث غيرها من الحمّيات من[8] غير أن يكون شيء[9] من الحمّيات سببا لحدوثها، ثمّ بعد[10] ذلك نذكر الأدواء على سبيل

<hr>

١٤ تشرك: تدرك DO

١ بألمها: ألمها D

٢ بريد: تدبّر B

٣ لأنّها: أنّها DOT

٤ باطن الجسد وظاهره: البدن وباطنه B ظاهر البدن وباطنه I

٥ والقوّى: -T

٦ الأرواح: + والقوّى النفسانية والأفعال الطبيعية B

٧ لأنّ: أنّ BO

٨ من...الحمّيات: -T

٩ شيء: شيا I شيء من: سائر B

١٠ بعد ذلك نذكر: نقوّي ذلك بذكر B نقفوا ذلك بذكر I نبدأ ذلك على ذكر O يقوي ذلك بذكر T

ما رتّبنا[1] في صدر كتابنا.

الباب الأوّل[2] في حمّى يوم

أقــول إنّ حمّـى يوم تتـولّـد عن حـرارة مـفـرطة[3] تسـخـن
الأرواح من غير مادّة ولا عفونة ولذلك لا تأخذ إلا يوما واحدا،
وأعني بالأرواح الروح الحـيـواني الذي هو ينبـوع[4] الحيـات
ومادّة[5] الحـرارة الغريزية والروح النفساني الذي هو ينبوع
الحسّ[6] والحـركـة والروح[7] الطبيـعي الذي هو ينبوع القوّى
الطبيـعيـة[8] الأربع أعني القوّة الجاذبة[9] والماسكة والهاضمة
والدافعة.

وهذه الحمّى تنقسم على ضـربين لأنّ منها مـا يكون هـي[10]
المرض نفسه ومنها ما يكون عرضا تابعا لمرض قد تقدّمه. فما

---

[1] رتّبنا: بيّنّا D

[2] الأوّل: + من المقالة السابعة BDO

[3] مفرطة: مفردة DIO

[4] ينبوع: مادّة T

[5] مادّة: وهذه O

[6] الحسّ: الحمى D الحسّ والحركة: -T

[7] والروح الطبيعي: -T

[8] الطبيعية: -O

[9] الجاذبة والماسكة والهاضمة: الحارة وهي الهاضمة والماسكة D

[10] هي: -D هو B من O

كـان منهـا هو¹ المرض نفسـه كـان² لـه³ أسـباب ثلاثة:
أحـدها أسـباب ظاهرة نظرا⁴ على الأبدان من خـارج مـثل
حرارة الشمس الصيفية والسموم والبرد الشديد والاستحمام
بالمياه التي لها قوّة على تجفيف ظاهر الأبدان وتكثيفها مـثل
المياه النطرونية والشبّية⁵ والكبريتية، والسبب الثاني إفراط
الحركة الجسدانية مثل⁶ التعب والنصب وإدمان المشي وما
أشبـه ذلك وإفراط الحركة النفسانية مـثل الحرد⁷ الشديد
وإدمان الفكرة في الهمـوم والأحـزان وسـائر همـوم النفس،
والسبب الثالث الإدمان على الأغذية الحارّة والأشربة المسخّنة
للدم ومـا شـاكل ذلك. فـأمّـا حمّى⁸ يوم التي هي عرض تابع
لمرض قد تقدّمها فمثل الحمّى التابعة لأورام الأرنبة⁹ وأورام
الإبط والعنق ومـا شـاكل ذلك. وذلك أنّ الدم الذي في الورم
إذا لبث فـيـه ولم ينحلّ سريعا حمي وتعفّن وأسـخن الروح

35

40

---

¹ هو: هذا B

² كان: فإنّ B

³ له: لها O

⁴ نظرا: تطوي B

⁵ والشبّية والكبريتية: -D

⁶ مثل: على T

⁷ الحرد: الحر DT الخزن O

⁸ حمّى يوم: الحمّى I

⁹ الأرنبة: الأزبنة B الأربية IT

الحيـواني واتّصلت حرارته بالقلب لاتّصـال[1] الشـريانات
بالقلب وحدث عن ذلك حمّى يوم، فـهذه جمل[2] أسبـاب حمّى
يوم.

فلنخبر الآن بخاصّة كل واحد[3] من تلك الأسباب وبرهانها
ونرتّب بعـقب[4] ذلك التـدبـير النافع لأصحـاب[5] هذه الحمّى
بإيجاز واختصار. فأقول إنّه يستدلّ على حمّى يوم العارضة
من حرارة الشمس بأنّ روس أصحابها تسخن وتكون أكثر
حـرارة من حـرارة[6] أبدانهم،[7] وذلك لوصـول وهج الشـمس
إلى أدمغتـهم ويكثر صداعـهم وتحمرّ[8] وجوههم وكثيرا[9] ما
يعرض[10] لهم زكام حارّ محرق للخياشيم.

فأمّا الحمّى التي تعرض من وهج السموم فإنّ حرارة أبدان
أهلها تكون أكثـر من حـرارة روسـهم[11] ويكون ظاهر أبدانهم

45

50

55

---

[1] لاتّصال: لاتّصالات O لاتّصال الشريانات بالقلب : T-

[2] جمل: O- تجعل D فهذه أسباب حمّى يوم: T-

[3] واحد: واحدة I

[4] بعقب: بعد O

[5] لأصحاب هذه الحمّى: B-

[6] حرارة: O-

[7] أبدانهم: أبدانهنّ I

[8] وتحمّر: وتحمى DO

[9] وكثيرا: وكثير BO

[10] يعرض: O-

[11] روسهم...حرارة: D-

ملتهبة جافّة من قبل أنّ حرارة السموم تنشّف رطوبة أبدانهم.

فـأمّا الحمّى التي تعرض من البرد والزمـهرير فـإنّ من دلائلـها أنّ ألوان أصـحـابها[1] تتـغيّـر ويزول عنها رونق الدم وحسنه وينتقل إلى لون الغبرة والكمودة ويبرد ظاهر أبدانهم وتجفّ وتقحل[2] ويجدون في روسهم مع[3] البرد ثقلا.

فـأمّا الذين[4] يعرض لـهم هذه[5] الحمّى من الاستـحـمـام بالمياه القابضة المجفّفة فإنّ جلودهم أجفّ وأقحل[6] من جلود من عرضت له هـذه الحمّى من البرد والزمهرير حتى أنّك إذا لمست جلود[7] أصحابها باليد وجدت[8] كأنّها قد نقعت[9] في نقيع العفص وقشر الرمّان زمانا. فإذا لبثت[10] يدك[11] على مـوضع من أبدانهم حـينا[12] حتى تسـخن جلودهم[13] بحرارة

---

[1] أصحابها: أهلها O

[2] وتقحل: وتنحل O

[3] مع: من D

[4] الذين: التي B الذي O

[5] هذه الحمّى: الحمّى BT حمّى O

[6] وأقحل: وأنحف DO

[7] جلود أصحابها: B- جلودهم صحابها O

[8] وجدت: وجدتها B

[9] نقعت: انتقعت O

[10] لبثت: لمست DO لبث I

[11] يدك: بيدك D

[12] حينا: -T

يدك¹ تحلّل من أبدانهم مـا كـان قـد احـتـقـن فـيـهـا لتكاثف
جلودهم واستحصافها² *ببخرات³ غريزية حارّة.⁴

فـأمّـا حمّى يوم العارضة من الأغذية والأشربة الحارّة فإنّ
ذلك الغـذاء يلهب الدم⁵ بحـرارته ويلهب الروح الطبيـعـي لأنّ
مـسكنه الكبد ومـركبـه الدم وتتّصل الحرارة بعد ذلك بالقلب
وتنتـشـر⁶ إلى جـمـيـع البـدن. ولذلك⁷ يكون البـول في
أصحـاب هذه الحمّى أكـثـر حمـرة منه⁸ في سـائر ضروب
حـمّى يوم لأنّ البـول⁹ مـائيـة⁹ الدم¹¹ ومـصـابّة¹² الأخـلاط
ولذلك يجدون في وقت منتهى الحمّى حرارة في أكبادهم.¹³

70

75

---

¹³جلودهم: أبدانهم O

¹يدك: أبدانهم T

²واستحصافها: واستلصاقها O واستحكانها D

³*ببخرات: بحرارة BO بخرات DIT

⁴حارّة: حادّة BI

⁵الدم: البدن I

⁶وتنتشر: وتبرز D

⁷ولذلك: + الدم Dˡ

⁸منه: فيه D

⁹البول: اللون O

¹⁰مائية: يأتيه I

¹¹الدم: -D

¹²ومصابّة: ومصبابة B وفضيلة D ومصالة IT

¹³أكبادهم: كبودهم DIT

فأمّا حمّى يوم العارضة من التعب الجسداني فإنّ أبدان
أصـحــابــهــا تكون ذابلة قــحلة' جــافّــة' ويجــدون في'
مـفاصلهم وهنا شــديدا وألما' قويا دائما ويكون عرقهم عند
منتهى حمّاهم دون العرق الحادث في سائر صنوف حمّى يوم.
وذلك أنّ هذه الحمّى إذا زالت رسومها وأخذت في الانحطاط
تحلّل من سطح البـدن نداوة شبـيهـة بنداوة الأبدان عند
خروجها من الحمّام. ومنهم من يعرق عرقا محمودا' فإن لم
يكن نداوة' ولا عــرق فــلا بدّ من' أن يكون بخــار كــثيــر'
يرتفع' من'' عمق البدن.

فأمّا حمّى يوم العارضة من الحرد والغضب فدليلها حمرة
وجوه أصـحــابـها وجحظ'' أعينهم'' وسرعــة حركتـها

'قحلة: نحلة O

'جافّة: -O

'في: + أبدانهن B

'وألما قويا دائما: دائما قويا B

'محمودا: شديدا T

'نداوة: ندا I

'من: -IO

'كثير: -I

'يرتفع: -B مرتفع O

''من: في B

''وجحظ: وشحط B

''أعينهم: عيونم O

وجفوف ١ أجفـانهم وقوّة مجسّتهم ٢ وعظمها وربّما اصفرّت
ألـوانهم واعـتـرتهم رعـدة. ويكون ذلك ٣ إذا خـالط ٤ الحـرد ٥
والغضب الفزع.

٩٠ فـأمّا حمّى يوم العارضـة من الغمّ أو من الهمّ فـإنّ أعين ٦
أصحابها تكون غائرة ساكنة وتقلّ نضارة ٧ وجوههم وتقبح
ألوانهم وتذبل أبدانهم وترقّ مجسّتهم وتحمرّ ٨ أبوالهم. وهذه
الدلائل قـد تعمّ ٩ من اهتمّ واغتمّ بنحـو من الأنحـاء وأقـرب ١٠
مـا يميّـز ١١ به ذلك أمـر ١٢ العينين، وذلك أنّ ١٣ العينين من
٩٥ صـاحب الهمّ والغمّ يكونان جـافّـتين. وأمّـا غـور ١٤ العينين

١ وجفوف أجفانهم: -D

٢ مجسّتهم: مجسّها T

٣ ذلك: كذلك O

٤ خالط: خلط B

٥ الحرد: الحدة D

٦ أعين: عيون DIO

٧ نضارة: نظارة BO

٨ وتحمرّ: وتحتدّ DIT

٩ تعمّ: تعرض D

١٠ وأقرب: وأكثر B

١١ يميّز به بذلك: يعتريه ذلك D يميّز ذلك T

١٢ أمر: من D

١٣ أنّ العينين: -T

١٤ غور: غوور BT غيور I

فـعـامّ' لجـمـيـع أصـحـاب هذه العـوارض أعني' الهمّ والغمّ
والسـهـر،' ويعـمّ جـمـيـعـهم أنّ' أبوالهم تكون أصبغ° صفرة
ويكون مع' من عـرضت له الحـمّى من غم من حدّة الحـرارة
أكثر' ممّا معـه من كثرتها . فإذا علم الطبيب سبب الحمّى
التي تأخـذ يومـا واحـدا واستـبـان له ذلك من الأعـلام
والدلالات^ التي° ذكـرنا فـيـنبـغـي عند ذلك أن يبـادر
بأصحابها'' إلى الحمّام.

فإن كانت الحمّى من حرارة الشمس والسموم فيدخلوا''
الحمّام عند سكون الحمّى'' وانقضاء سورتها ولا يطيلون
المكث فيه ويفرش بين أيديهم الرياحين الباردة المسكّنة للبخار

100

105

'فعامّ لجميع: فيعمّ جميع O

'أعني: من O

'والسهر: -D

'أنّ: في O

°أصبغ: أصبغ D أسبغ I أشبع T

'مع: -O

'أكثر: بأكثر T

^والدلالات: والدلائل DO

°التي...الحمّام: -T

''بأصحابها : + بالدخول B

''فيدخلوا: فيدخلون O

''الحمّى: -I

مـثـل الورد والبنفسج والخـلاف` وورق الـبـزرقطونا وترطب
خياشيهم في كلّ وقت بدهن البنفسج ودهن النيلوفر وتمسح
أصـداغـهـم بدهن الورد مـضـروبا` بالخلّ ويصبّ على
روسهم` بعد انكسار الحمّى مـاء قد طبخ فيه نوّار بنفسج
وبابونج وذلك إن لم يكن بهم زكام ولا صداع، فـإن كان في
روسـهم` شيء من الامتـلاء فليـحـذروا° ذلك ويقتصروا`
على الانكباب على بخاره فقط. ويسقوا` مـاء الرمّانين مع
سكّر طبـرزد ويتّخذون من الأشـربة الجلاب وشراب البنفسج
وشـراب الورد وشـراب الإجّـاص ويغـذّوا° بلباب الخـبـز
المغـسـول مع سكّر طبـرزد ويغذّوا° أيضا`` بالقرع والرجلة
ولبّ القثّـاء وقلوب الخسّ ويمصّ`` الرمّان. ويتـغـذّون`` بعد

110

115

` والخلاف: والذلاف B

` مضروبا: المضروب D مضروب I

` روسهم: رؤوسهم B

` روسهم: رؤوسهم B

° فليحذروا: فليحذرون I

` ويقتصروا: ويقتصرون BDI

` ويسقوا: ويسقون BDO

° ويغذّوا: ويغذّون BD

° ويغذّوا: ويغذّون BDO

`` أيضا: -B

`` ويمصّ: ومصّ D

`` ويتغذّون: ويغذّون D

زوال الحـرارة بـالدرّاج والفـراريج بماء الرمّـانين أو بماء
الحصرم.

فإن كانت الحمّى من البرد والزمـهرير فينبغي إذا نضج
الفضل وانهزمت الحمّى أن تنزل¹ أرجلهم² في ماء قد طبخ
فيـه بابونج ومـرزنجوش وشبثّ ونمام وينكبّون على بخاره
ويدخلون بعد ذلك حمّاما عذبا ويكون مقامـهم في³ هواء⁴
الحمّام أكـثـر من المقام في الأبزن وذلك أنّ هواء⁵ الحمّـام
يعرق⁶ الأبدان ويحلّل رطوباتها ويفتح مسامّها . ومن كان من
أصحاب هذه الحمّى به نزلة من⁷ برد فليحـذر دخول الحمّـام
أصـلا إلا بعـد نضج⁸ النزلة⁹ وانحـلالهـا، ويشمّـون¹⁰
روائح¹¹ ذكية مثل المرزنجوش والياسمين والخيري وما أشبه

120

125

---

¹تنزل: يتركوا D

²أرجلهم: رجلهم O

³في هواء الحمّام: فيه D

⁴هواء: هذا O

⁵هواء: هذا D

⁶يعرق: يفرق T

⁷من...النزلة: D¹

⁸نضج: نضوج I

⁹النزلة: العلّة I

¹⁰ويشمّون: ويشتمّون O

¹¹روائح: روائحا I رائحة O

ذلك ويدثّرون¹ بالثياب ويجعلون بالقرب منهم نار جمر تمنع
برد الهواء من الوصول إليهم وتطلى² روسهم³ بالأدهان
التي تسخّن إسخانا معتدلا مثل دهن البابونج أو دهن الشبثّ
أو دهن الخيري أو دهن السوسن وما أشبه ذلك.

فإن عرضت هذه الحمّى⁴ من الاغتسال بالمياه القابضة
المجفّفة فينبغي أن يمنعوا⁵ أصحابها من دخول الحمّام إلا
بعد انقضاء سورة الحمّى وانهزامها وبعد أن تنزل أرجلهم في
الماء قد طبخ فيه بابونج وشبثّ ومرزنجوش وما شاكل⁶ ذلك،
ويؤمروا⁷ بالانكباب على بخار الماء وإذا دخلوا الحمّام
فيدلكوا⁸ أبدانهم فيه دلكا رفيقا⁹ ويصبّوا¹⁰ عليها ماء
عذبا فاترا، فإنّ ذلك يليّن جلودهم ويفتح مسامّها¹¹.

130 (margin)
135 (margin)

---

¹ويدثّرون: ويتدثّرون O

²وتطلى روسهم: وتنطل أبدانهم T

³روسهم: رؤوسهم B رعوسهم I

⁴الحمّى: الحمّايات T

⁵يمنعوا: يمنع BO + أيضا DT

⁶شاكل: أشبه T

⁷ويؤمروا: ويؤمرون BD ويؤمروا بالانكباب: ويدمنون الانكباب O

⁸فيدلكوا: فيدلكون BDO

⁹رفيقا: خقيقا D

¹⁰ويصبّوا: ويصبّون BDO

¹¹مسامّها: مسامّهم BOT

ويحذروا١ الدهن في الحمّام فإنّه يسدّ مسامّ الأبدان ويحصر
البخارات في باطنها. والرياضة المعتدلة من٢ أحمد الاشياء
في علاج٣ هذه الحمّى لأنّها٤ تحلّل الأبدان وتفتح
مسامّها٥ وتحلّل البخار٦ المنحصر٧ فيها. وبالجملة٨
فينبغي لأصحاب هذه الحمّى أن يحذروا كلّ ما يبرد الجلد
ويقبضه ويسدّ مسامّه، ويستعملوا٩ الأغذية السريعة
الانهضام ويسقوا١٠ شراب السكّر ممزوجا١١ بالماء،

فإن عرضت هذه الحمّى من الأغذية الحارّة فينبغي أن
يسقى العليل سكنجبين سكّري أو ماء الرمّانين ممزوجا١٢
بالجلاب أو بالسكّر١٣ الطبرزد ويسقى بعد ذهاب الحمّى من

140

145

---

١ ويحذروا: ويحذر T

٢ من: في D

٣ علاج: مداوات I

٤ لأنّها ... فيها: -T

٥ مسامّها: + وتفتح بخارها I

٦ البخار المنحصر: البخارات المنحصرت(!) D

٧ المنحصر: المحتصر I

٨ وبالجملة: وفي الجملة B

٩ ويستعملوا: ويستعملون BDO

١٠ ويسقوا: ويسقون BD

١١ ممزوجا: ممزوج IT

١٢ ممزوجا: ممزوج I

١٣ بالسكّر: ماء السكّر D

أقرصـة الطبـاشيـر أو أقرصة الكافـور مع شـراب بنفسـج
أو شـراب الورد ويضمّـد الكبـد بالطحلب أو بالرجلة ولعـاب
البزرقطونا وقشـور القرع أو بصندل ودقيق شعير وشيء من
كـافـور مـعـجـون بماء الورد. ويكون الغـذاء الرجلة والهندباء
والسـرمق والقـرع، ويمزج المـاء عند العطش بشـراب
البزرقطونا أو بشراب الرمّانين.

فإن عرضت هذه الحمّى من التعب الجسداني فينبغي أن
يلتمس لهم الهدوء والراحة وتمرخ أبدانهم تمريخا رفيقا
بدهن بنفسـج أو دهن ورد أو دهن نيلوفـر. ويدخلوا
حمّامـا معتدلا في هوائه ومائه ولا يطيلوا الجلوس فيه،
وتمرخ أبدانهم عند خروجهم من الماء العذب الحارّ بدهن
بنفسـج أو دهن الورد ويسقـوا مـاء الرمّانين مع شـراب

150

155

160

---

١ أقرصة: أقراص B

٢ أقرصة: أقراص B

٣ ويضمّد: ويكمّد D

٤ ويمزج: ويمزجون B + لهم D ويمزوا(!) I ويمزجوا T

٥ الجسداني: -D

٦ تمريخا: مرخا BO

٧ بنفسج...بدهن: -D

٨ ويدخلوا: ويدخلون O

٩ هوائه ومائه: مائه وهوائه I

١٠ العذب: -B

١١ ماء الرمّانين مع: -B

البنفسج أو شراب الإجّاص أو شراب الجُلاب. ويتغـذّون بالأغـذية المرطبـة[1] لأبدانهم مـثل الفـراريج ولحوم الجـداء والسمك النهري[2] وما أشبه ذلك.

فإن عرضت[3] هذه الحمّى من إفراط الحركة النفسانية فينبغي أن يقابل السـبب المؤذي للنفس[4] المتعب[5] لهـا بما ضادّه[6] ونفاه[7] مـثل أن يقابل الغيظ والغمّ والغضب بتسكين النفس وتلذيذها بالكلام وبالفعـال[8] مـثل أن يتـشـاغلوا[9] بضروب من الملاهي المطربة المفرّحة والنظر إلى الأشياء التي ترتاح لهـا[10] النفس مـثل الرياحين الخضـرة والوجـوه[11] المقبـولة. ويلتمس فيهم مع إصلاح النفس بما ذكرنا من[12]

165

170

---

[1] المرطّبة: O- الرطبة D

[2] النهري: الطري B

[3] عرضت: + لهم D + له T

[4] للنفس: لليبس O

[5] المتعب: المنفت(!) O

[6] ضادّه: يضادّه D ضادّده B يضاده O

[7] ونفاه: وينفيه DO ونافاه I

[8] وبالفعال: والفعل B وبالفعل D

[9] يتشاغلوا: يشتغلوا O يشاغل B يشاغلوا T

[10] لها: إليها I

[11] والوجوه: + النظرة O

[12] من: IT-

إصلاح البدن بما يرطبه¹ ويزيل عنه يبسه العارض له مثل
أن يدخلوا حمّاما عذب الماء معتدل الهواء ويتمرّخوا² عند
خروجهم من الماء الفاتر بدهن بنفسج أو دهن نيلوفر ولا
يكثروا الغمز³ في الحمّام فإنّ ذلك يزيدهم يبساً وجفافا .
ولذلك⁵ يؤمرون⁶ بترك الجماع والحركة ويتغذّون⁷
بحسو⁸ الشعير والقرع والرجلة والبقلة اليمانية.⁹ وإذا
زالت الحمّى يغذّوا¹⁰ بالدرّاج والفراريج ولحم الجداء.
ويشربون¹⁰ شرابا معتدل المزاج¹¹ ويشمّوا الصندل والكافور
والورد والبنفسج والآس ويمصّوا¹² ماء الرمّانين¹³ وماء

١٧٥

---

¹يرطبه: يطربه DI

²ويتمرّخوا: ويتمرّخون I

³الغمز: التعرق D المقام O

⁴يبسا: عسا B

⁵ولذلك: وكذلك O

⁶يؤمرون: يؤمروا IT

⁷ويتغذّون: بعد(!) D ويتغذّوا I

⁸بحسو: + المعمول من B

⁹اليمانية: الحمقا D

¹⁰ويشربون: ويشربوا T

¹¹المزاج: -O

¹²ويمصّوا: ويعطوا D

¹³الرمّانين: الرمّان DT

١

العنب الشتوي ويسقوا¹ ماء الدلاع مع السكّر الطبرزد. 180
وبالجملة يجتنبون الأشياء الميبّسة² ويستعملون³ الأشياء
المرطبة ويقدّر⁴ ذلك فيهم على قدر قوّة العليل وسنّه ومزاجه
الطبيعي وعادته والوقت من السنة والبلد وسائر ما أشبه ذلك.

ومن عرضت له هذه الحمّى من ورم⁵ الأرنبة⁶ فينبغي أن
يعالج ذلك الورم ويعمل في إنحلاله ويداوى⁷ معه العفن⁸ 185
الذي بسببه حدث الورم، ثمّ يدبّرون بمثل ما قدمنا. فهذا
القول في دلائل حمّى يوم وعلاجها على طريق الاختصار.

الباب الثاني في الحمّى المحرقة

أمّا الحمّى المحرقة المدعوة باليونانية قوسوس⁹ فحمّى 190
يكون معها عطش شديد دائم وحرارة مطبقة مؤذية مقلقة¹⁰

---

¹ ويسقوا: ويسقون T

² الميبّسة: الموجسة(!) B

³ ويستعملون: ويستعملوا IT

⁴ ويقدّر: ويقرر O

⁵ ورم: وجع B

⁶ الأرنبة: الأزبنة B

⁷ ويداوى: ويراد(!) B

⁸ العفن: العضو B + والعضو I العضل O

⁹ قوسوس: فوسوس B

¹⁰ مقلقة: معلقة O

للطباع¹ مهيّجة لها² على مصارعة المرض ومجاهدته من ابتدائه لحدّة³ العنصر⁴ المولّد لها وحرافته لأنّ تولّدها عن عنصر حادّ ناري صفراوي قد اجتمع في أفضية العروق المجاورة للقلب وبخاصّة عروق فم المعدة وتقعّر⁶ الكبد وتجويف الرئة.

والأعراض اللازمة لهذه الحمّى الحرارة المطبقة والعطش الدائم الذي لا يفتر. وإنّما⁷ صارت الحرارة في الحمّى المحرقة مطبقة من قبل أنّ المرار الذي عنه تتولّد في داخل العروق، وإنّما صلبت الحمّى ودامت لأنّ أكثر المرار المولّد لها في العروق المجاورة للقلب. ولمّا كان المرار المولّد لهذه حمّى مخصوصا بعروق فم المعدة وتقعّر⁸ الكبد كما بيّنا اشتدّ العطش ودام⁹ ولم¹⁰ يفتر.

وأصناف الحمّى المحرقة صنفان أحدهما خالص صعب

195

200

---

¹للطباع: للطبيعة B

²لها: له B

³لحدّة: بحدّة B محدث(؟) D فحدّة T

⁴العنصر: العضو O

⁵حادّ: حارّ IO

⁶وتقعّر: ومقعّر O

⁷وإنّما: وربّما O

⁸وتقعّر: وقعر B وبعروق D ومقعّر O

⁹ودام: -OT

¹⁰ولم: ولا B

والآخر مشوب سهل. فأمّا الخالص الصعب فإنّ تولّده عن¹
المرار الأصفر الخالص² الحدّة والحرافة³، وأكثر تولّده في
الأحداث والشبّان⁴ وفي من كان مـزاجـه بالطبع حـارّا⁵
حريفا وبخاصّة في زمان⁶ الصيف لأنّ الزمان⁷ الصيفي
مقوٍّ لهذه الحمّى بالطبع وزائد فيها. وأمّا السهل المشوب فمن
مرار أصفر⁸ يخالطه رطوبة عذبة أو بخار عذب. ولمّا كانت
هذه الحمّى عظيمـة الخطر مضـمّنة بالخـوف⁹ وجب على
المتطبّب¹⁰ أن يحذرها من الابتداء ويستعمل فيها الوقوف¹¹
على معرفة أوقات المرض الأربعة، أعني الابتداء والصعود
والمنتهى¹² والهبوط¹³ ويستعمل في كلّ وقت منها ما يجب

205

210

---

¹عن...تولّده: I-

²الخالص: + الصعب B

³والحرافة: والحرارة B

⁴والشبّان: والشباب BT

⁵حارّا: حادّا T

⁶زمان: زمن IT

⁷الزمان: الزمن IT

⁸أصفر: صفراويّ B

⁹بالخوف: بالجوف B

¹⁰المتطبّب: الطبيب D

¹¹الوقوف: الوقت(!) O

¹²والمنتهى: والانتهاء OT

¹³والهبوط: والانحطاط D

استعماله.

فإذا رأى في ابتداء المرض أنّ الطبيعة محتاجة إلى ما يحرّك الفضول ويستفرغها فينبغي أن يسقي العليل ماء التمر الهندي والإجّاص والعنّاب مع[1] لبّ خيار شنبر قصبي وترنجبين خراساني وبنفسج مربّى وشراب الإجّاص وما أشبه ذلك. فإن فات الطبيب تحريك الطبيعة في ابتداء المرض لعائق[2] منع من ذلك مثل ضعف القوّة وامتناع احتمالها للاستفراغ أو لفجاجة الفضل وغلظه فينبغي له[3] أن يحذر ذلك غاية الحذر في صعود المرض لأنّه إن فعل ذلك تحيّرت الطبيعة لشغلها[4] بالدواء وحارت وخلت[5] عن تدبير المرض أصلا. ولكن إذا فات[6] تحريك الطبيعة من ابتداء المرض فينبغي أن يعين الطبيعة على حفظ القوّة بالغذاء السريع الانهضام المحمود الجوهر مثل حسو الشعير المحكم الصنعة أو لباب الخبز المغسول بالماء البارد[7] غسلات.

وقد ذكر جالينوس في كتابه في البحران كيف ينبغي

---

[1] مع...ذلك: -B

[2] لعائق: -I

[3] له: -OT

[4] لشغلها: وشغلها B

[5] وخلت عن: -BDO وحلت I

[6] فات: كان D

[7] البارد: -B

للطبيب¹ أن يكون تغـذيتـه للمـرضى² في العلل الحـادّة³ 230
فـقـال: الأعـراض في تدبير غذاء المريض⁴ ثلاثة الأعراض:
أحدها مـقـدار القوّة من المرض⁵ والآخر مـقـدار مدّة⁶ المرض
والثالث كيفية المرض. فأمّا⁷ مقدار القوّة من المرض فيما⁸
يحتاج إليه من حفظها إذا كانت هي المقاومة⁹ للمرض ولذلك
قد ينيل¹⁰ الغذاء للمريض كثيرا¹¹ إذا¹² خفنا على القوّة أن 235
تخـور¹³ من غـيـر أن يلتـفت إلى الوقت.¹⁴ وأمّـا مـقـدار¹⁵

---

¹للطبيب: للطبع B

²للمرضى: للمريض DO للمرض I

³الحادّة: الحارّة DI

⁴المريض: المرض I

⁵المرض: المريض I المرض...من T-

⁶مدّة: O¹

⁷فأمّا: أو O

⁸فيما: فما B

⁹المقاومة: المفارقة D

¹⁰ينيل الغذاء للمريض: يميل المرض للغذاء B يقبل المريض الغذاء D ينيل
المريض الغذاء I ينيل الغذاء O

¹¹كثيرا: أكثر O

¹²إذا خفنا: خوف B

¹³تخور: O- يجوز T

¹⁴الوقت: المرض I

¹⁵مقدار: + قوة I

مدّة¹ المرض فيحتاج إلى النظر فيه حتى يقدّر الغذاء بحسب
قرب² منتهى المرض وبعده، فإن كان المنتهى قريبا استعملت
اللطافة المفرطة جدّا إلى أن يأتي³ المنتهى⁴ ولم⁵ يغذّ⁵
بشيء.⁶ فإن كان المنتهى بعيدا⁷ غذوت أوّلا فأوّلا قليلا
قليلا إلى أن ينتهي المرض على التدريج. وأمّا بحسب كيفية
المرض⁸ فمن قبل أنّ جميع المحمومين في المثل يحتاجون
إلى التدبير الرطب، وما كان من الحمايات مع نقصان من
البدن فالحاجة⁹ فيه إلى الغذاء أكثر حتى لربّما أغذينا¹⁰ فيه
في وقت الحمّى.

وما كان من الحمّيات مع فضول في¹¹ البدن فينبغي أن
يحذر فيه كثرة الغذاء ولا¹² يكون إلا في أوقات الفترات بين

240

245

---

¹مدّة: قوّة O

²قرب منتهى: قوّة O

³يأتي: O¹

⁴ولم: -B

⁵يغذّ: بعد BI يغذّى OT

⁶بشيء: -B

⁷بعيدا: + غذاء B

⁸المرض: المريض O

⁹فالحاجة: فإنّ الحاجة I

¹⁰أغذينا: غذينا IT

¹¹في: -I

¹²ولا...الغذاء: -I

نوائب الحمّى، ويحذر الغذاء في جميع أوقات نوبة الحمّى[1].

فإن[2] لم يكن بين نوائب الحمّى أوقات فترات وسكون منها[3]

كـان وقت[4] الغـذاء وقت انحطاط نوبة الحمّى، فـإن لم يكن

للحمّى انحطاط واحتجنا أن نغذّي المريض[5] اخترنا له الوقت

الذي كان من عادة ذلك المريض أن يغتذي فيه وهو صحيح

وبخاصّة أوقات طيّبة من النهار باردة رطبة[6] مثل الغدوات

لنشـاط الطبيـعـة في ذلك الوقت ولطافة[7] النسـيم وانكسار

الحمّى لمقاومة برد السحر لحرارتها وقمعه[8] لحدّتها. فهذا

قـول حكيم الطبّ وفيلسوفـه جالينوس[9] في كيـفـيـة غذاء

المرضى[10] في العلل[11] بألفاظه نصّا[12]. قـد ذكرناه لعظيم

فائدته وجليل منفعته في مثل هذا الموضع من هذا الكتاب.

---

[1] نوبة: غيبة B

[2] فإن لم يكن بين نوائب: فإن كان بين أوقات I

[3] منها: فيها D

[4] وقت: -O

[5] المريض: العليل B

[6] باردة رطبّة: I- رطبة T

[7] ولطافة: في لطافة I

[8] وقمعه: -B

[9] جالينوس: -I

[10] المرضى: المرض DO المريض I

[11] العلل: العليل O

[12] نصّا: -B

ولمّا كـانت هذه الحمّى أعني المحـرقـة من ابتـدائهـا إلى
انقضائها في حال شدّة وصعوبة وجب أن نقتصر فيها على
التدبير اللطيف مثل حسو شعير ولباب الخبز المغسول بعد أن
يلقى عليه سكّر طبرزد مسحوق، ويعطون في بعض الأوقات
مـا يسكّن حـرارة المعـدة مـثل مصّ الرمّان[1] الإمليـسي[2]
والعنب الشتـوي ولبـاب الفقّـوص[3] ويستخـرج لهم لعاب
البزرقطونا في ماء الدلاع[4] ويسقوه[4] ويسقون شراب بنفسج
أو شـراب الإجّـاص أو شراب البزرقطونا أو شراب الجلاب
الرفيع. ويسـقى[5] بالعشي وزن درهمين بزرقطونا مغسـولة
بالمـاء البـارد ودرهم بزر رجلة أو طين أرمني مع مـاء الرمّان
الحلو[6] قـدر[7] خمسـة أواق وعشـرة دراهم سكّر سليـماني
مسحوق أو شراب بنفسج.

وإن احتـاج[8] إلى الغذاء[9] بعد أن يعطى بالغدوات ماء[10]

---

[1] الرمّان: + الحلو I

[2] الإمليسي: المليسي DIOT

[3] الفقّوص: العنوس(!) T

[4] ويسقوه: IO-

[5] ويسقى: + العليل D

[6] الحلو: -BT

[7] قدر...مع ماء الرمّان أو: -B

[8] احتاج: احوج IT

[9] الغذاء: + يغذى I

[10] ماء ...مغسولا مع ماء الرمّان الحلو أو: -T

الشـعير مع مـاء الرمّـان الحلو[1] أو[2] مع شـراب البنفسـج فإن
لم يقم به ذلك فيعطى فتات[3] مـغسـولا مع ماء الرمّان الحلو أو
سـويق الشـعير مـغسـولا[4] بالماء البارد غسـلات مع سكّر
طبرزد ويكون[5] ذلك في وقت انكسـار الحمّى قليلا ويتّقون ذلك
ويحذروه[6] في وقت سـورة المرض إلا[7] عند الضرورة.

فإن كان في الطبيعة تعذّر وامتنـاع ليّنـاها قبل سـورة المرض
بأن يؤخـذ من مـاء القرع المشـوي في عجين شـعير بإحكام
نصف رطل ويمرس فيه ترنجبين خراسـاني وبنفسج مربّى من
كلّ واحد عشـرة دراهـم ويصفّى ويلقى على الصفو أوقية من
شـراب الإجّـاص السـاذج ويسـقاه. فإن احتجت إلى تقويته[8]
قليلا فـزد فيه وزن خمسـة دراهـم لبّ خيـار شـنبر منقّى[9] من
قصبـه وحبّه. أو يسـقى مـاء نقيـع الإجّاص الأسـود والتمـر
الهندي مع شـراب بنفسج وترنجبين خراسـاني.

---

[1] الحلو: O-

[2] أو...الحلو: I-

[3] فتات: لباب الخبز B فتيت O

[4] مغسولا: مغسول IT

[5] ويكون ذلك: T-

[6] ويحذروه: ويحذرونه IOT

[7] إلا عند...المرض: T-

[8] تقويته: سهاله(!) D

[9] منقّى من قصبه وحبّه: D-

285 فإن أجابت الطبيعة بذلك وإلا فاستعمل شيافا ١ متّخذا من

ورق بنفسج ونطرون من كلّ واحد وزن نصف مثقال وسقمونيا

وزن نصف درهم وحضض وزن مـثـقـال تدقّ الأدوية ويحلّ ٢

الحضض في ماء حارّ ويعجن به الدواء ويعمل منه فتل أمثال

البلّوط ويمسح بدهن بنفسج ويستعمل.

290 فإن أجابت الطبيعة بذلك وإلا فاتّخذ لهم حقنة بماء العلّيق

وماء السلق وماء النخالة من كلّ واحد أوقيتين وشراب بنفسج

أو شـراب الإجّاص ودهن بنفسج من كلّ واحد أوقية ودرهم

نطرون مـسـحـوق ويخلط ٣ ويفتر ويستعمل. ويرطب المعدة

ويبرد حرّها بلعاب البزرقطونا مع ماء الرمّان أو مع مـاء

295 الدلاع ويسـتـعـمـل ٤ خلاء ٥ المعـدة في وقت سـورة المرض ٦

من الغـذاء إلا ٧ أن تدعـو ٨ الضرورة مـثـل أن يخاف على

القوّة بأن تضعـف في وقت المجـاهـدة بين الطبيعـة والمرض

فـقـوّيها ٩ بشيء من مـاء الشعـير أو الفتات ١٠ المغسول ولا

---

١ شيافا متّخذا: شياف متّخذ I

٢ ويحلّ: وينحل D

٣ ويخلط: -O

٤ ويستعمل: + ويرطّب B + على D

٥ خلاء: خلل I جلاء T

٦ المرض : الحمّى O

٧ إلا أن تدعو الضرورة: إذا دعت الضرورة إلى ذلك O

٨ تدعو: تدعوا I تدعوه T

٩ فقوّيها: فقوّها DI

يعطى من ذلك إلا مقدار ما يحفظ¹ القوّة فقط.

300 فإن عرض للعليل صداع فيؤخذ دهن الورد ويضرّب بخلّ²
خمر أو بماء الرجلة أو بماء جرادة القرع وتمسح به الجبهة
والأصداغ ويؤخذ أيضا دهن بنفسج أو دهن نيلوفر ويسعط
منه ويمزج³ بماء الورد مـبـرّدا⁴ في لعاب الـبـزرقطونا
ويحمّل⁵ على الجبهة والأصداغ، وتدخل⁶ القدمان والساقان
305 فـي مـاء حـارّ⁷ عـذب وتغمـز بدهن بنفسج وتشدّ الساقان
بعصائب، ويحمّل⁸ على الجبهة والأصداغ ضماد متّخذ من
صندل محكوك ودقيق شعير وورق ورد معجون بماء الورد أو
بماء الطحلب أو بماء جرادة القرع أو بماء الرجلة أو بلعـاب
البزرقطونا.

310 فإن كان بالعليل سهر وأرق فيزاد في هذا الضمـاد بزر⁹

---

¹الفتات: العناب D

¹يحفظ: + به O

²بخلّ خمر: بالخلّ الجيّد I

³ويمزج: ويمرخ I

⁴مبرّدا: مبرّد I

⁵ويحمّل: ويعمل D

⁶وتدخل..والأصداغ: -I

⁷حارّ: -O

⁸ويحمّل: ويعمل D

⁹بزر خسّ: ترنجبين B

خسّ وبزر خشـــخـــاش ويعـجن بماء الخس ويشمّ١ دهن
النيلوفر ودهن البنفسج. فإن عرض للعليل جفاف في فمه٢
وخشونة في لسانه فيتمضمض بلعاب البزرقطونا ولعاب حب
السـفـرجل ويلقى عليـه شيء من سكّر طبرزد ودهن بنفسج.
فإن كان في اللسان سواد فيخلط مع هذه اللعابات ماء الورد
ودهن الورد ويدلك به اللسـان أو يمسك في٣ فـمــه٤ مـاء
الرمّان الحلو مخلوط بدهن الورد.

فـإن عـرض للعليل خـفـقـان٥ يسـقى لعـاب البـزرقطونا
المستخرج بماء القثّاء مع شراب الجلاب أو شراب الرمّان
أو٦ شـراب الحصـرم أو شـراب حمّـاض الأترنجّ. ويحـمّل٧
على معدهم٨ ضماد متّخذ من الصندلين ودقيق الشعير
مـعـجـون بماء الورد، أو يؤخـذ الطحلب والرجلة ولعـاب
البـزرقطونا وجـرادة القرع فـيخلط بماء الورد ودهن الورد
ويحمّل٩ على المعـدة والكبـد في وقت خـلائـها من الغذاء.

---

١ ويشمّ: ويشتمّ I

٢ فمه: فيه I

٣ في: -O

٤ فمه: فاه B فيه IO

٥ خفقان: جفاف B

٦ أو شراب الحصرم: -O

٧ ويحمّل: ويعمل D

٨ معدهم: مقدمتهم O

٩ ويحمّل: ويعمل D

ويسقون سويق الشعير مغسول غسلات بعد أن يلقى عليه ٣٢٥

سكّر طبرزد أو جلاب أو رمّان[1] حلو ويغذون[2] بقرع معمول

بماء الحصرم وماء حمّاض الأترنجّ وقضبان الرجلة[3]

ويغذون[4] بعدس مقشور مطبوخ مع قرع وسكّر طبرزد وماء

الحصرم أو شيء من خلّ، ويفرش بين يدي العليل الآس

والخلاف والورد ويرشّ على الريحان الماء الحين[5] بعد الحين. ٣٣٠

وكثيرا ما يعرض في هذه الحمّى التي كلامنا فيها البرسام

أو السعال اليابس[6] أو الغشي أو اليرقان فإن[7] عرض

ذلك[8] فيؤخذ علاجه والتدبير النافع له من الباب الذي

أفردنا[9] له[10] في[11] هذا الكتاب.

الباب الثالث[12] في حمّى الغبّ ٣٣٥

---

[1] رمّان: ماء الرمّان IT

[2] ويغذون: ويغذوا T

[3] الرجلة: السفرجل D

[4] ويغذون: -D ويغذوا IOT

[5] الحين بعد الحين: المرّة بعد المرّة D

[6] اليابس: -O

[7] فإن عرض ذلك: -O

[8] ذلك: -I

[9] أفردنا له: أوردناه B فردنا له I

[10] له: + ذلك D

[11] في: من DO

[12] الثالث: + من المقالة السادسة B

وحمّى الغبّ تسمّى باليونانية اطريطاوس وهي بالعربية
المثلّثة وإنّما تتولّد عن كيموس صفراوي إذا استحال وتعفّن
إلا أنّه متى[1] كانت تلك العفونة خارجة من العروق والأوردة
أحدثت حمّى الغبّ ذات النوائب التي تأخذ وتترك، وعرض
معها برد وقشعريرة ورعدة. ومتى كانت تلك العفونة داخل
العروق والأوردة أحدثت إمّا حمّى غبّ دائمة وإمّا حمّى
قوسوس أعني المحرقة.

فإن قال قائل بماذا توافق الحمّى المحرقة حمّى الغبّ
الدائمة[2] وبماذا[3] تخالفها قلنا له أمّا اتّفاقهما ففي أنّهما
جميعا يحدثان عن الخلط الحارّ الصفراوي وفي أنّهما داخل
العروق والأوردة[4] وفي أنّهما دائمتان وأمّا الفرق بينهما ففي
المواضع[5] التي يجتمع المرار المولّد للحمّى فيها[6]، وذلك أنّ
الالتهاب العارض في الحمّى المحرقة يكون في العروق
المجاورة للقلب وبخاصّة عروق فم المعدة والكبد والرئة أكثر
منه[7] في عروق سائر البدن لأنّ المادّة هناك أكثر كما[8] بيّنا

---

[1] متى كانت تلك: متكاثف وتلك O من تلك(!) D

[2] الدائمة: I-

[3] وبماذا تخالفها: I-

[4] والأوردة: والأوراد I

[5] المواضع التي: الموضع الذي BD

[6] فيها: فيه D

[7] منه: منها I

[8] كما: فيما D

340

345

350

آنفا، وفي حمّى الغبّ الدائمة يكون الالتهاب العارض منها في جملة عروق[1] البدن مثله في الأوعية المجاورة للقلب.

وقـد يسـتـدلّ على حمّى الغبّ بثـلاثة دلائل: أحـدهـا من الأشياء الطبيعية[2] والثاني من الأشياء التي ليست بطبيعية والثالث من الأشياء الخارجة من[3] الطبيعة. فأمّا الاستدلال عليها من الأشياء الطبيعية فهو أنّ أكثر[4] تولّدها فيمن كان مـزاجـه حـارًّا يابسـا وسنّه من اثنين[5] وعشرين الى خمسـة وثلاثين سنة وبخـاسّة إذا كـان بدنه نحيـفـا ومسـامّ بدنه متحلّلا[6]. وأمّا الاستـدلال عليها من الأشياء التي ليست بطبيعية وهو أنّ أكثر تولّدها في زمان[7] الصيف وبحاصّة إذا كانت طبيعـة الهواء الحـاضر[8] حـارّة يابسة ومزاج البلد أيضـا كذلك وتصرّف[9] العليل في حـال[10] صحّـتـه في الكدّ والتعب والنصب. وأمّا الاستدلال عليها من الأشياء الخارجة

355

360

---

[1] عروق: I-

[2] الطبيعية...والثالث من الأشياء B-

[3] من: عن D

[4] أكثر: O-

[5] اثنين وعشرين: ابنا عشرين B خمس وعشرين D اثنى عشر O

[6] متحلّلا: متخلخلا B متخلخلة DIT

[7] زمان: O-

[8] الحاضر: I-

[9] وتصرّف: ويعرف I

[10] حال: جل O

عن الطبيعة أعني بذلك الأعراض المتولّدة عن طبيعة العنصر
المولّد للحمّى التي هي للمريض¹ أعراض وللطبيب دلائل
وعلامات وهي أنّه لمّا كان تولّد هذه الحمّى عن العنصر الحارّ
الصفراوي المجاور للأعضاء الحسّاسة وجب أن تتقدّمها
قشعريرة صعبة لها نخس كنخس الإبر والشوك لأنّ الصفراء
بحدّتها إذا مرّت بالأعضاء الحسّاسة التي لم تألفها وانصبّت
عليها لدغتها بحرافتها² وأحدثت فيها نخسا وتولّد من ذلك
قشعريرة، وإنّما يكون هذا إذا كانت المادّة خارجة عن العروق.

وقد يخصّ³ هذه الحمّى أيضا ويلزمها القيء المرّي
والإسهال المصبوغ بالمرّة وبخاصّة في⁴ النوبة الثالثة
والرابعة وتكون أبوالهم حمراء نارية لطيفة. ومن خاصّة هذه
الحمّى شدّة الحرارة والفوران ونخس في الكبد لممازجة⁵
المرّة⁶ الدم. وأكثر ما يمكث⁷ دور هذه الحمّى إذا كانت⁸
خالصة اثنتي⁹ عشرة ساعة وسكونها ستّة¹⁰ وثلاثين ساعة

365

370

375

---

¹للمريض: للمرض I

²بحرافتها: بحرارتها O

³يخصّ: تختصّ OT

⁴في: ب– O في..ومن خاصّة: –B

⁵لممازجة: للمازجة I

⁶المرّة الدم: المرّة الصفرا للدم D بالمرّة بالدم I المرّة للكبد O الكبد للدم T

⁷يمكث: يدوم I

⁸كانت: + في I

⁹اثنتي عشرة: اثني عشر BDI اثني عشرة O

وأكثر ما تكون أدوارها إذا كانت خالصة سبعة أدوار وهي[1]
أربعة عشر يوما فإن زادت نوبتها على اثنتي[2] عشرة ساعة
وأدوارها على سبعة أدوار فليست بخالصة. وإذا لم تكن
خالصة وامتزجت بغيرها جازت هذا الحدّ وطال لبثها حتى
أنّها ربّما ابتدأت في الخريف وتركت في الربيع.

وهذه الحمّى أعظم صنوف[3] حمّيات العفن خطرا
وأقربها[4] من الخوف، ولذلك يجب على المتطبّب أن يحذر فيها
من استعمال الأشياء الحارّة خوفا من[5] أن ترقى المرّة
الصفراء بحدّتها إلى الدماغ فيحدث فيه ورما ويصير العليل
إلى البرسام فيكون ذلك أعظم لخطر الحمّى وأشدّ لخوفها.
وذلك أنّ المرّة الصفراء لطيشها وحدّتها وخفّتها لا تحتمل
خطاء[6] العليل ولا جهل الطبيب ولكن ينبغي أن ينظر الطبيب
في ابتداء العلّة فإن كانت قوّة العليل حسنة مساعدة والأخلاط
هائجة متحرّكة عند ذلك الطبيعة بمطبوخ متّخذ من
الإجّاص والتمر الهندي ونوّار البنفسج والهليلج الأصفر
ويمرس فيه لبّ خيار شنبر وترنجبين ويسقى منه على

<hr />

[1] ستّة: سبعة D

[1] وهي...أدوار: O

[2] اثنتي عشرة: اثني عشر BDI اثني عشرة O

[3] صنوف: -I

[4] وأقربها من الخوف: وأقرب خوفا O

[5] من: -I

[6] خطاء: -D

أرقام الأسطر: 380، 385، 390

مقدار¹ القوّة والسنّ. ويسهل أيضا بماء الرمّانين المدقوقين
بشحمهما مع سكّر سليماني أو يسقى من النقوعات أو
الأشربة التي ذكرنا في كتابنا هذا² أنّها تسهل المرّة
الصفراء وتقمع حدّتها وتسكّن غليانها، ويحذر³ استعمال
ذلك غاية الحذر في يوم النوبة لئلا يدخل على الطبيعة ما
يشغلها عن مصارعة المرض.

ويعطى في أيام النوائب ماء الرمّانين قدر نصف رطل مع
أوقية⁴ شراب بنفسج أو شراب إجّاص أو يسقى ماء⁵
القرع المشوي مع⁶ سكّر طبرزد. فإن كانت الحرارة قوية
والعطش⁷ شديد فيقتصرون على البزرقطونا وزن مثقالين مع
ماء الرمّانين وشراب الجلاب ويحذرون غاية الحذر أن يأخذوا
في وقت النوبة شيئا من الغذاء ولا قبل النوبة بثلاث ساعات.

فإن كانت نوبة الحمّى تأتي بالغداة فيقتصرون على شراب
الجلاب أو شراب الرمّان أو شراب الإجّاص إلى أن تنقضي
نوبة الحمّى فيأخذوا بعد انقضاء النوبة حسو الشعير المحكم

---

¹ مقدار: قدر O

² هذا: -I

³ ويحذر: + العليل O

⁴ أوقية: + من O

⁵ ماء: -I

⁶ مع: فيسقى منه من D

⁷ والعطش: والغشي D

الصنعة ويتناولون في آخر النهار' لباب خبز مغسول بالماء

مرّات' مع شيء من سكّر طبرزد مسحوق.

وإن كانت الطبيعة متعذّرة وفاتهم في ابتداء المرض أخذ'
الدواء المانع' وعاقهم' عن ذلك' مثل هواء فاسد أو
ضعف قوّة أو غير ذلك فينبغي أن يعطوا في أيام الترك من
الترنجبين الخراساني والبنفسج المربّى من كلّ واحد وزن
عشرة دراهم ولبّ خيار شنبر منقّى' من حبّه وقشره وزن
خمسة دراهم، يمرس ذلك في ماء عذب حارّ مرسا جيّدا أو
يمرس في ماء القرع المشوي ويصفّى ويزاد فيه أوقية من'
شراب الإجّاص' الساذج ويشرب بالغداة.

ويأخذون في يوم النوبة لعاب البزرقطونا بماء الرمّانين
وشراب البنفسج أو شراب الإجّاص أو سكر سليماني، فإن
أجابت الطبيعة واعتدلت بهذا التدبير وإلا فيؤخذ'' لهم

' النهار: الليل T

' مرّات: دفعات B

' أخذ: أخذوا T

' المانع: النافع I

' وعاقهم: عاقهم BDT

' عن ذلك -BT

' منقّى من حبّه وقشره: -DI من حبّه وقشره O من حبّه وعيدانه T

' من شراب: -O

' الإجّاص.. وشراب: -D

'' فيؤخذ: يتّخذ BIT

شياف¹ من نوّار بنفسج وسقمونيا ونطرون وسكّر أحمر
وحضض أو يستعمل لهم حقنة تتّخذ من إجّاص وعنّاب
ومخيطا ونوّار بنفسج وشعير مقشور وماء النخالة² وماء³
السلق ودهن بنفسج وسكّر وبورق ويدبّر بإحكام ويستعمل
بلطافة.

ويجعلون تدبيرهم في اليوم السادس مثل تدبيرهم في
أيام⁴ النوائب ليأتي اليوم السابع وأبدانهم على⁵ غاية
الخلاء⁶ والنقاء وتنفرد الطبيعة بمصارعة⁷ المرض وتلطيف
المادّة من غير أن يشغلها عن ذلك بأخذ غذاء ولا دواء.

فإن شكى العليل في وقت السورة عطشا وجفافا في لهواته
وحلقه فيتجرّع لعاب البزرقطونا المستخرج بماء القثّاء⁸ مع
شيء من دهن بنفسج ويستخرج اللعاب⁹ بماء الدلاع أو بماء
الرمّانين ويتمضمض¹⁰ بلعاب البزرقطونا ولعاب حبّ

425

430

¹شياف من: شراب T

²النخالة: النخلة B

³وماء السلق: -O

⁴أيام: أوّل O

⁵على: في O

⁶الخلاء و-: -D

⁷بمصارعة: بمشاركة I

⁸القثّاء...بماء: -O

⁹اللعاب: اللعابات IT

¹⁰ويتمضمض بلعاب البزرقطونا: -O

435 السـفرجل ودهن البنفسج، ويمزج لهم أيضـا المـاء¹ بشـراب
الإجّـاص أو شـراب الجـلاب أو شـراب البنفسـج أو شـراب
البزرقطونا على ما دبّرناه وذكرناه في باب السعال.

فـإذا زال عن العليل² الالتـهـاب وانكسـرت حـدّة الحمّى
واشتكى لدغا في معدته فيعطى لباب خبز مغسول مع سكّر
440 طبرزد ويغـذوا³ من البـقـول بالسرمق⁴ والبـقـلة اليمـانيـة
والخـيـار والقـرع والخسّ يطبخ لهم بالماش والكزبرة الرطبـة
ودهن اللوز ويكون هذا⁵ بعد زوال⁶ الحمّى والكرب.

فإن عرض لهم صداع فينبغي أن يحـمّلوا⁷ على الجبين
والأصـداغ دهن ورد أو دهن بنفسج مـضـروبا⁸ بالخلّ،
445 ويرطبـون الخيـاشيم بدهن النيلوفر أو⁹ دهن بنفسج أو دهن
حبّ القـرع. فـإن غلب اليبس على أدمغـتـهـم وعرض لهم
البرسـام فيسعطون بأحد هذه الأدهان مع لبن امرأة ترضع

---

¹أيضا الماء: inv. I

²العليل: العلة D

³ويغذوا: ويغذون B ويغذى D

⁴بالسرمق: كالسرمق BI السرمق T

⁵هذا: الغذاء D

⁶زوال: B¹

⁷يحمّلوا: يجعل D يحملون I

⁸مضروبا: مضروب I

⁹أو دهن بنفسج: T-

جارية ويحلب على روسهم¹ الألبان ويصبّ عليها ماء قد طبخ فيه خشخاش وخسّ² أو بزره ونوّار بنفسج وورق³ البزرقطونا وتدخل أرجلهم في ماء حارّ⁴ عذب وتغمز بدهن البنفسج ويجعل بين أيديهم رياحين باردة.

فإن جاءهم في اليوم السابع قيء أو إسهال طوعا عن⁵ فعل الطباع⁶ فينبغي أن يترك ما احتملته القوّة⁷ ويسقون ما يسكّن حرّ المعدة ويقطع العطش مثل شراب الحصرم أو شراب الرمّانين أو شراب التفّاحين أو شراب الورد أو الورد المربّى أو شراب الكمّثرى، وينقع لهم في الماء طباشير وصندل وبزر رجلة.

فإن أفرط الإسهال وخفنا على القوّة أن تسقط بادرنا بعلاج ذلك وحبسه⁸ بربّ الآس وربّ السفرجل وأقراص الطباشير المعمولة ببزر الحمّاض وما أشبه ذلك من الأدوية الباردة القابضة على سبيل ما ذكرنا في باب الإسهال. وكذلك إن عرض لهم سحج أو غشي أو يرقان فيعالج ذلك من موضعه

450

455

460

---

¹روسهم: -D

²وخسّ : -T

³وورق: O¹

⁴حارّ عذب: inv. I

⁵عن: من T

⁶الطباع: الطبيعة I الطبائع O

⁷القوّة: الطبيعة B

⁸وحبسه...فيعالج ذلك: -D

ألذي أفـردنـاه[1] لذكـر[2] ذلك العـارض على حسـب مـا يراه الطبيب في كلّ[3] واحد[4] من المرضى.

465

الباب الرابع[5] في الحمّى المتولّدة من الدم وتسمّى باليونانية سونوخوس[6]

إنّ الدم لمّا كان أعدل العناصـر طبـعـا وألذّهـا[7] طعمـا وأقربها من مزاج الإنسـان ألّفته الطبيعة لذلك وجعلته مادّة

470

لغذاء[8] الأبدان[9] وقوامها وصيّرته جوّالا مـعـها في جميع البدن لتستمدّ منه الأعضاء إذا كان منه تغذيتها وبه قوامها وتقويتها . فإن زاد الدم في كمّيته[10] واستحال وتغيّر عن كيفيته[11] شنأته[12] الطبيعة وخلت عن تدبيره كما يشنأ[13] المرء

---

[1] أفردناه: أفردنا له OT

[2] لذكر ذلك العارض: -T

[3] كلّ: -O

[4] واحد: وقت(!) D

[5] الرابع: + من المقالة السابعة B

[6] سونوخوس: سوخوس I سونوخس T

[7] وألذّها طعما: -O

[8] لغذاء: لضد(!) D

[9] الأبدان: البدن I الأبدان I¹

[10] كمّيته: كيميته BO

[11] كيفيته: طبيعته I

[12] شنأته: شنته IO نسيته T

ولده إذا خرج عن طاعته وهو أحظى الناس عنده وأخصّهم
به[1] فيبقى فجّا غير منهضم[2] وخرج عن حدّ الاعتدال
475 واستحال وعفن وتولّدت عن عفونته الحمّى التي تسمّى
باليونانية سونوخوص[3] أيّ حمّى دائمة وهي المطبقة وذلك أنّ
الدم على مجرى الطباع داخل[4] العروق والأوراد وهي
سبله[5] وطرقه إلى جميع البدن.

وقد أقام جالينوس في كتابه في فصول الحمّيات البراهين
480 الواضحة في أنّ أصناف حمّى العفونة صنفان: منها[6] ما
يكون من عفونة الأخلاط داخل[7] العروق والأوراد و منها ما
يكون من عفونة الأخلاط خارج[8] العروق وأنّ الحمّى إنّما
تكون دائمة إذا كانت العفونة داخلة[9] العروق وإنّما[10] يكون

---

[13] يشنأ: سنسى T

[1] به: فيه O

[2] منهضم: نضيج I

[3] سونوخوس: سوناخوس IO سونوخس T

[4] داخل: + في BT

[5] سبله: سببله (= سبيلة؟) O

[6] منها: منهما I

[7] داخل...الأخلاط: -B

[8] خارج: + عن I

[9] داخلة: داخل BDO

[10] وإنّما...العروق: -O

لها فترات إذا كانت العفونة¹ خارجة من العروق. وقد يتولّد
عن الدم الخـالص حمّى حـارّة² إذا حـمي والتـهب داخل
العـروق والأوراد من غيـر أن تلحـقه عفونة ولا فـساد، ومن
خاصّة³ هذه الحـمّى أنّ الربو تابع⁴ لهـا دائمـا في أكـثر
الحـالات لأنّ تولّدها⁵ عن مـا بيّنّا من الدم النقي وهذا الدم
أكـثر قوّته في القلب والرئة ولذلك لقّبت الأوائل⁶ هذه الحمّى
بالحرارة الربوية⁷ من قبل أنّ أكـثر أسبـاب الربو إنّمـا يكون
عن حرارة الصدر⁸ والقلب والرئة.

والفرق بين الحمّى المتولّدة عن عـفونة الدم وبين الحمّى
المتولّدة عن غليان الدم وفورانه أنّ الحمّى المتولّدة عن عفونة
الدم مـعـها نتن في البول ونبض العروق⁹ فيـها مـختلف لأنّ
انقـباض العـرق¹⁰ إلى¹¹ داخل اسـرع من انبـساطه¹² إلى

485

490

495

---

¹العفونة: الحمّى I

²حارّة: حادّة BIT

³خاصّة: خاصّية O

⁴تابع: نافع O

⁵تولّدها: + يكون O

⁶الأوائل: -D

⁷الربوية: + الدمية I

⁸الصدر والقلب: inv. I

⁹العروق: العرق IT

¹⁰العرق: العروق O

¹¹إلى داخل: الداخل I داخل T

خارج من قبل مبادرة الطبيعة إلى إخراج البخارات الدخانية المتولّدة عن العفونة بسرعة. والحمّى المتولّدة عن غليان[1] الدم خلية[2] من هذه الأعراض.

وقد يتقدّم حمّى الدم علامات تنذر بحدوثها قبل ظهورها مثل[3] كسل[4] وثقل[5] الأعضاء وامتـلائهـا وحمـرة اللون وحرارة سطح[6] البدن. ويتبعها علامات بعد[7] ظهورها مثل الصـداع والالتـهـاب وثقل الرأس وتورّم الصدغين وجحظ[8] العينين وقلّة[9] العطش وكثرة[10] السبات وخيالات حمـر ترى نصبة العينين وقوّة النبض وسرعته وحمرة البول الشبيهة بحـمـرة الأرجـوان. وكثيرا[11] مـا يعـرض مـع[12] هذه الحـمّى

500

505

---

[12]انبساطه: انبساطها O

[1]غليان: -I

[2]خلية: خلو BDIT

[3]مثل: من T

[4]كسل: التكسير BIT التكسّل O

[5]وثقل: وضعف O

[6]سطح: تطبخ(!) D

[7]بعد ظهورها: تنذر بحدوثها قبل ظهورها O

[8]وجحظ: + في DOT

[9]وقلّة ...العينين: -B

[10]وكثرة: و- D

[11]وكثيرا: وكثيرة O وكثير I

[12]مع: في I

الورشكين' والجدري.

ولمّا كانت هذه الحمّى متولّدة' عن عفونة الدم داخل العروق والأوراد كما بيّنا فينبغي أن نبادر قبل صعود المرض وبلوغه سورته فننظر في صحّة' القوّة ومساعدة السنّ والمزاج والزمان وطبيعة الهواء الحاضر والعادة. فإن كانت هذه الدلائل ممكنة وبخاصّة صحّة القوّة' فصدنا العليل° وأخرجنا له' من الدم على قدر' الكفاية.

فإن كان ابتداء المرض بعقب طعام كثير أكله المريض وهو مجتمع في جوفه' فينبغي أن يؤخّر' الفصد إلى اليوم الثاني وما بعده حتى تقوى الطبيعة على هضم الطعام وإنضاجه وإخراج فضله من الأمعاء والبطن. فإن لم تفعل ذلك الطبيعة فعلنا نحن ذلك بالتدبير المليّن للبطن.

فإن لم يساعدنا من هذه الدلائل التي ذكرنا'' إلا صحّة

'الورشكين: الزرشكين B + والحصبة D

'متولّدة: المتولّدة O

'صحّة القوّة: صحّته B

'القوّة: البدن D

°العليل: + الأكحل B

'له: -B

'قدر: مقددار I

'جوفه: معدته I

'يؤخّر: يؤخذ آخر D

''ذكرنا: ذكرناها T

القوّة فـقط أمـرنا بإخراج الدم من الحـجـامـة عـوضـا من¹
الفصد. وإن سـاعـدتـنا كلّ الدلائل إلا أنّ² القـوّة ضـعـيـفـة
وجب³ أن نحـذر إخـراج الدم بفـصـد أو حجـامـة لأنّ صـحّـة
القوّة وثبـاتهـا⁴ هي المجـاهـدة⁵ للمرض. فـينبغـي لنا أن
نراعـي القوّة دائمـا ونتـثـبّت⁶ فيـهـا⁷ حسـنا ونسـتـعـمـل
استقصاء النظر في صحّتها وثباتها على مـقـاومة⁸ المرض
قبل أن نتـقدّم⁹ على إخراج الدم.

فإن تعـذّر إخـراج الدم في ابتـداء العـلّة لوجـه من الوجوه
فينبغـي¹⁰ أن يحـذر ذلك غاية الحـذر في صعـود المرض ومنتهاه
وإن ألفـينا¹¹ القـوّة صـحـيـحـة حسـنة لأنّ في¹² هذين الوقتين
من المرض لا يوثق بصـحّـة القوّة لشـغـلهـا بمجـاهـدة المرض

520

525

530

¹من: عن I

²أنّ: بأنّ T

³وجب...القوّة: -B

⁴وثباتها: ومياها(!) D

⁵المجاهدة: المخلفة B

⁶ونتثبّت: وتثبت DT

⁷فيها: فينا D

⁸مقاومة: وفارقة D

⁹نتقدّم: يقدم DT نقدم I

¹⁰فينبغي أن يحذر: فينبغي لنا أن نحذر DT

¹¹ألفينا: لقينا B نظرنا D

¹²في: -BD

ومصارعته. لكن ينبغي لنا أن نستعمل تطفئة الدم وتسكين
حدّته بلعـاب البـزرقطونا، بماء الرمّانين وشـراب البنفسج
وشراب الإجّاص السـاذج.[1]

فإن كان في الطبيعة امتناع فيؤخذ لذلك تمر هندي منقّى
وزن[2] عشرة دراهم وإجّاص عشرون عددا ونوّار بنفسج وزن
ثلاثة مثاقيل، يطبخ ذلك في رطلين ماء حتى يبقى نصف رطل
ويصفّى من غـير مـرس ويحلّ في ذلك[3] الصـفـو ترنجبين
خراسـاني ولبّ خيـار شنبر منقّى من كلّ واحد وزن عشـرة
دراهم ويصفّى أيضا ويشرب.

فإن كان في الصـدر علّة مـتـقـدّمـة أو عارضـة مع الحمّى
فـيؤخـذ لذلك عشـرون[4] حبّة عنّاب و نوّار بنفسج وبزر رجلة
من كلّ واحد وزن خمسة دراهم، فيطبخ مثل الأوّل ويحلّ فيه
بنفسج مربّى وترنجبين خراساني ولبّ خيار شنبر منقّى[5] من
كلّ واحد وزن سـتّـة دراهم ويصـفّى ويشـرب. ويعطون من[6]
الغذاء ما كان لطيفا سريع الانهضام محمود الجوهر مثل[7]

---

[1] الساذج: I-

[2] وزن...بنفسج: T-

[3] ذلك: B-

[4] عشرون حبّة عناب: عناب عشرين حبّة I

[5] منقّى: DI-

[6] من الغذاء: الأغذية B

[7] مثل: + صفو BI

حسو الشعير المحكم الصنعة أو فتات¹ مغسول بالماء²
غسلات. فإن لم يكن الدم حادًّا³ فيجب أن تليّن الطبيعة في
الابتداء بما فيه مع التبريد تلطيف، بمثل ماء القرع المشوي
بعد أن يحلّ⁴ فيه ترنجبين خراسانيّ ولبّ خيار شنبر
ويشرب.⁵

فإن أجابت الطبيعة باستعمال ما قدّمنا وإلا فتتّخذ لهم
شيافات أو حقن ليّنة متّخذة من عنّاب ومخيطا ونوّار بنفسج
وشعير مقشور⁶ وسكّر ودهن بنفسج⁷ وما أشبه ذلك. فإن
عرض لهم صداع فيستعملون ترطيب الخياشيم بدهن بنفسج
أو دهن نيلوفر ويؤخذ دهن الورد فيضرّب بخلّ ويحمّل⁸ على
الجبهة والأصداغ. أو⁹ يخلط دهن الورد بماء الورد أو بماء
الخلاف¹⁰ أو بماء الحصرم أو بماء الرجلة ويحمل على الجبين

550

555

---

¹فتات: + خبز DT

²بالماء غسلات: .inv I

³حادًّا: حارًّا O حادًّا مريا B حارًّا مريا I

⁴يحلّ: يحلب(!) T

⁵ويشرب: -T

⁶مقشور: مقشر O

⁷بنفسج: + أو دهن نيلوفر O

⁸ويحمّل: ويعمل D

⁹أو...والأصداغ: -T

¹⁰الخلاف: الجلّاب IO

والأصداغ.‏ وتنزل‏[1] اليدان والرجلان في ماء قد طبخ فيه بابونج وبنفسج يابس وتشدّ الساقان بعصائب.‏

560 فإن لم يسكن الصداع وكان الصدر بريئا‏[2] من النوازل والسعال فيحلب على الرأس ألبان النساء وألبان الأتن ويغسل بماء قد طبخ فيه شعير‏[3] مقشور ونوّار بنفسج وبابونج ويسعطون بدهن بنفسج ودهن نيلوفر ويضمّد الرأس بضماد متّخذ من ماء الرجلة وجرادة‏[4] القرع ولعاب البزرقطونا 565 ودقيق الشعير وماء‏[5] الورد وما أشبه ذلك.‏

فإن عرض لهم غمّ والتهاب فيسقون لعاب البزرقطونا المستخرج بماء القثّاء أو بماء الرمّانين ويسقون أيضا ماء الدلاع مع سكّر طبرزد أو بالجلاب. فإن عرض لهم سبات‏[6] يحول بينهم وبين فتح أعينهم فينبغي‏[7] أن يمنع‏[8] من أن 570 يقرب الرأس‏[9] بشيء‏[10] مما وصفنا من الأخبصة‏[11]

‏[1] وتنزل:‏ ويترك T

‏[2] بريئا من النوازل:‏ يربا من النوار(!) B

‏[3] شعير...بنفسج و–:‏ –D

‏[4] وجرادة:‏ وبرادة T

‏[5] وماء الورد:‏ O[1]

‏[6] سبات:‏ شيء B

‏[7] فينبغي:‏ + لنا T

‏[8] يمنع:‏ يمتنع DIO

‏[9] الرأس:‏ الناس O للرأس D

‏[10] بشيء:‏ شيئا DT

والأدهان ويقتصر على غمز القدمين[1] في ماء البابونج ونوّار بنفسج ودهن[2] بنفسج وملح جريش[3] ويمسح الجبين والأصداغ بماء البابونج ونوّار البنفسج ويطعموا[4] ماء الرمّان[5] المرّ مع فتات[6] الخبز المحكم الصنعة المغسول بالماء مرّات.

575

فإن عرض لهم خفقان ضمّدنا المعدة بضماد متّخذ من صندل وورق ورد ودقيق شعير وشيء من كافور معجون بماء الورد أو بماء الرجلة أو بماء القرع، ويتجرّعوا[7] ماء الورد ويسقوا[8] شراب الرمّان أو شراب الجلاب.

580

فإن عرض لهم رعاف فينبغي أن يحمّل على الجبين والأصداغ الضماد الذي وصفنا[9] للخفقان ويسعطوا[10] بماء البلح الأخضر أو ماء الطلع مع شيء من كافور ودهن

---

[11] الأخبصة:الأخبهية(!) D الحقنات O

[1] القدمين: الساقين B

[2] ودهن: بدهن IT ودهن..ونوّار البنفسج: -O

[3] جريش: جراش B

[4] ويطعموا: ويطعمون BD

[5] الرمّان المرّ: الرمّانين O

[6] فتات: لباب DIOT

[7] ويتجرّعوا: ويتجرّعون BD

[8] ويسقوا: ويسقون BD

[9] وصفنا: وصفناه O

[10] ويسعطوا: ويسعطون B ويسقون D

ورد ويعالجون¹ بالتدبير الذي ذكرنا عند نعتنا² للرعاف.

فإن احتجنا في آخر هذه الحمّى إلى ما يسكّن ويطفئ
بقاياها من البدن فإنّا نستعمل عند ذلك أقراصا³ جرّبناها
في تسكين حمّى الدم وتحليل الفضل بلطافة وتزيل الوهج
والحرّ وهذه صفتها: يؤخذ طباشير أبيض وصندل أصفر
محكوك وبزر رجلة وربّ السوس من كلّ واحد وزن مثقالين
ولبّ بزر القثّاء ولبّ بزر البطّيخ ولبّ حبّ القرع من كلّ واحد
وزن درهمين وكثيراء بيضاء وصمغ عربي ونشاستج من كلّ
واحد وزن درهم وكبابة وكافور من كلّ واحد وزن دانقين، يدقّ
ذلك وينخل ويعجن بلعاب البزرقطونا ويعمل من ذلك أقراص
وزن كلّ قرص مثقال ويجفّف في الظل ويسقى منها واحدة⁴
بماء القرع المشوي أو ببعض الأشربة الباردة. وإن أريد⁵ أن
يكون معجونا⁶ فيزاد فيه وزن أربعة مثاقيل سكّر طبرزد
ويعجن بالجلاب ويسقى منه وزن مثقالين فإنّه⁷ بديع عجيب
وينفع من الورشكين والحصبة⁸ والجدري.

585
590
595

---

¹ ويعالجون: ويعالج BIOT

² نعتنا: -O تعينا B تعب(!) D بعثتة(!) I

³ أقراصا: أقراص I

⁴ واحدة: واحد BD

⁵ أريد: أراد B

⁶ معجونا: معجون I

⁷ فإنّه: + نافع B

⁸ والحصبة: والحصبا BIT

الباب الخامس[1] في حمّى الربع

فأمّا حمّى الربع[2] فإنّها تتولّد عن[3] عفونة المرّة السوداء
فإن كانت المرّة السوداء المتعفّنة[4] داخل العروق والأوراد
أحدثت[5] حمّى الربع الدائمة[6] فإن كانت خارجة من العروق
والأوراد أحدثت[7] حمّى الربع الدائمة[8] ذات النوائب. وإنّما
سمّيت حمّى الربع لأنّها تأخذ في كلّ أربعة أيام مرّة ومقدار
نوبتها أربعة وعشرون[9] ساعة وتركها ثمانية وأربعون[10]
ساعة.

وقد يستدلّ على هذه[11] الحمّى بالثلاثة[12] دلائل التي
يستدلّ بها على حمّى الغبّ، أعني من الأشياء الطبيعية

___

[1] الخامس: + من المقالة السابعة B السادس O

[2] فإنّها: فانما B

[3] عن: من D

[4] المتعفّنة: + في B

[5] أحدثت...والأوراد: -T

[6] الدائمة..وإنّما سمّيت حمّى الربع: -D

[7] أحدثت: أورثت B

[8] الدائرة: الدائمة I

[9] وعشرون: وعشرين I

[10] وأربعون: وأربعين I

[11] هذه...يستدلّ بها على: -T

[12] بالثلاثة: بثلاث B بالثلاث O

والأشياء[1] التي ليست بطبيعية والأشياء الخارجة من
الطبيعة. فأمّا الاستدلال عليها من الأشياء الطبيعية فهو أنّها
أكثر ما تعرض في من كان مزاجه باردا يابسا وسنّه كهلا[2]
وبخاصّة متى[3] كان البدن[4] نحيفا جافًا مدمجا[5] وعروقه
ضيّقة خفية. وأمّا[6] الاستدلال عليها من الأشياء التي ليست
بطبيعية فإنّها[7] يستدلّ[8] عليها بطبيعة الفصل من السنة
إذا كان خريفا ومزاج الهواء الحاضر إذا كان باردا يابسا
وطبيعة البلدة إذا كانت كذلك. وأمّا الاستدلال عليها من
لأشياء الخارجة من[9] الطبيعة فهو أن هذه الحمّى تعرض
لأصحابها في[10] ابتداء كلّ نوبة من نوائبها[11] عند ابتداء
عفونة المادّة *ببرد[12] شديد متعب للبدن مفتّت للعظام وذلك أنّ

610

615

---

[1] والأشياء...الأشياء الطبيعية: -D

[2] كهلا: مكتهلا T

[3] متى: من D

[4] البدن: بدنه D

[5] مدمجا: -D مدعجا T

[6] وأمّا...خريفا: -O

[7] فإنّها: فإنّه I فإنّا B

[8] يستدلّ: نستدلّ B

[9] من: عن I

[10] في ابتداء كلّ نوبة: كينوبة(!) D

[11] نوائبها: قرابتها(!) D

[12] *ببرد: برد MSS

المرّة السوداء التي عنها تتولّد هذه الحمّى لبردها وغلظها إذا
انصبّت إلى الأعضاء الحسّاسة أثقلتها[1] وأوهتها[2] ورضّتها
وتكون ألوان أصحابها مائلة إلى الكمودة وجلودهم قحلة
جافّة.[3] وهذه الحمّى مخصوصة بوجع الطحال وصلابته
ويكون البول في ابتداء هذه الحمّى أبيض رقيقا مائيا. فإذا
انقضت الحمّى[4] ولطفت المادّة ورقّت[5] صار البول أسود.

ولـمّا[6] كانت هذه الحمّى تتولّد عن[7] عفونة مرّة سوداء
خالصة وهي الباردة اليابسة وتتولّد[8] عن مرّة سوداء متولّدة
عن[9] احتـراق الأخـلاط وتشيّطهـا[10]، أعني بالأخـلاط الدم
والمرّة الصفراء والبلغم، وجب[11] أن يميّز[12] كلّ واحدة[13] منها

---

[1] أثقلتها : بقلتها(!) D

[2] وأوهتها : وأوجعتها B وأوهنتها DT

[3] جافّة : يابسة D

[4] الحمّى : -O

[5] ورقّت...الحمّى : -T

[6] ولـمّا : وإنّما DO

[7] عن : من DO

[8] وتتولّد : + أيضا O

[9] عن : من O

[10] وتشيّطها : ويبسها O

[11] وجب : فوجب D

[12] يميّز : نصير (؟) I

[13] واحدة : واحد DIOT

بخاصّتها' المميّزة لها' ممّا' سواها' ليرطب' كلّ
صنف منها ما يلائمه من التدبير' والعلاج.'

وإن تبيّن لنا بالدلائل التي ذكرنا أنّ تولّد هذه الحمّى من
عفونة مرّة سوداء خالصة فينبغي أن ندبّر العليل بالأشياء
المنضجة السريعة الانحدار مثل ماء الهندباء وماء الرازيانج
وماء الكرفس، يؤخذ من جميعها نصف رطل بعد أن يغلى
ويصفّى ويلقى عليه أوقية من شراب سكنجبين عسلي أو
شراب العسل المدبّر بالأفاويه، أو يحلّ فيه ورد مربّى عسلي
ويشرب أو يسقى مطبوخ الأصول أو شراب الأفسنتين.

وتستفرغ المادّة بالقيء رويدا رويدا ويستدعى' العرق
بدهن البابونج أو بدهن الشبثّ أو بدهن الفوذنج النهري ولا
يستفرغ البدن في ابتداء' المرض استفراغا عنيفا. وإذا
أخذت الحمّى في الانحطاط وظهرت علامات النضج
والانهضام استفرغنا عند ذلك المرّة السوداء بالحقن

' بخاصّتها: بخاصّيتها O بخاصّته DIT

' لها: له DIOT

' ممّا: من I

' سواها: سواه DIOT

' ليرطّب: ليرطّب ل- B فنرطّب O لترطيب T

' التدبير: التبيد T

' والعلاج: والصلاح D

' ويستدعى: ويستفرغ O

' ابتداء: استبراء B

وبالأدوية¹ التي² تسهّل هذا الخلط، وسقينا³ العليل في
هذا الوقت أقراص الغافت وأقراص الراوند وأقراص
الآنيسون وأقراص اللك على النسخ التي⁴ قدّمنا ذكرها في
المقالة الخامسة من هذا الكتاب.

ويستعمل معها من⁵ الأشربة مثل شراب الإذخر وشراب
الفوذنج ومطبوخ الأصول، وقد يؤخذ في آخر هذه العلّة
الترياق⁶ المعروف بالفاروق والجوارش المعمول بالكمّون.
وينبغي⁷ أن يحذر استعمال⁸ هذه الأدوية في الصيف
والبلد⁹ الحارّ وسنّ¹⁰ الشباب وإنّما تستعمل في الشتاء وفي
البلدان الباردة وفي سنّ الشيخوخة وفي¹¹ من الغالب على
مزاجه البرد. ويمنع أيضا من استعمال الأشياء المبرّدة¹²

---

¹وبالأدوية: والأدوية I

²التي تسهل هذا: المسهلة لهذا D

³وسقينا: واسقينا OIT

⁴التي: الذي O

⁵من: + الأدوية و− O

⁶الترياق: الدرياق O الترياق المعروف بالفاروق: ترياق الفاروق D

⁷وينبغي أن يحذر: ويحذر I

⁸استعمال: + مثل IT

⁹والبلد: والبدن B وفي البلد I

¹⁰وسن: وفي سن I

¹¹وفي من: ومن I

¹²المبرّدة: الباردة I المبرّدة I¹

لأنّها تفجّج١ المادّة وتمنع من النضج فيصير ذلك سببا٢ 655
لطول مدّة المرض.

فإن كان قد تقدّم هذه الحمّى الربعية حمّى غبّ وكان العليل
شابًّا نحيفا ومزاجه صفراويا وبوله أشقر ناريا وعطشه
شديدا وأرقه٣ كثيرا والزمان مع ذلك صيفا وطبيعة الهواء
الحاضر حارّة يابسة علمنا من هذه الدلائل أنّ الحمّى تولّدت 660
عن احتراق مرّة صفراء. فينبغي عند ذلك أن يعالج العليل في
الابتداء بما يبرّد ويلطّف مثل ماء الرمّانين والسكنجبين
السكّري٤ وحسو٥ الشعير بماء الرمّانين والسكنجبين.٦

فإن كان في الطبيعة امتناع فليّنها٧ بماء الإجّاص
والترنجبين والبنفسج المربّى، أو يؤخذ من٨ ماء الهنداء وماء 665
الرازيانج مغلّى٩ مصفّى ويمرس١٠ فيه لبّ خيار شنبر منقّى

---

١ تفجّج: تفجّ T

٢ سببا: ميتا B

٣ وأرقه: وأراقه T

٤ السكّري وحسو الشعير بماء الرمّانين والسكنجبين: - T

٥ وحسو الشعير: - B

٦ والسكنجبين: - D

٧ فليّنها: فنلينها O فلتسهل I

٨ من: - B

٩ مغلّى: منقّى B

١٠ ويمرس: ممروس D

وترنجبين[1] ويشرب، فان لم تجب[2] الطبيعة بذلك أمرنا العليل[3] باستعمال[4] الحقن المسهلة. فاذا[5] أخذت المادّة في النضج وخفّت حركتها وانتقالها من مكان[6] إلى مكان فعند ذلك يسقى مطبوخا[7] يسهل المرّة الصفراء المحترقة من غير عنف مثل مطبوخ الإجّاص والتمر الهندي والترنجبين وما أشبه ذلك.

ويحـذر[8] ذلك قـبل نضج المادّة ويمصّـوا[9] الرمّانين[10] والعنب الشتوي ويغذوا[11] بالماش مع البقلة اليمانية أو مع السرمق. ويصبّون[12] على أبدانهم في آخر العلّة بعد انكسار الحمّى ماء[13] فاترا أو ماء[14] قد طبخ فيه بابونج وإكليل الملك

---

[1] وترنجبين: + خراساني B

[2] تجب: تجيب B

[3] العليل: -T

[4] باستعمال: أن يستعمل I

[5] فاذا: وإن I

[6] مكان إلى مكان: موضع إلى موضع O

[7] مطبوخا: مطبوخ I

[8] ويحذر: وتحدث T

[9] ويمصّوا: ويمضغ B ويمتص D ويمصّون I ويمصّ T

[10] الرمّانين: الرمّان T

[11] ويغذوا: ويغذون I

[12] ويصبّون على أبدانهم: ويضع على يديه O

[13] ماء فاترا: بماء فاتر I

ونوّار بنفسج ويتمرّخون بشراب مضروب بدهن بنفسج[1].

هإن تقدّم هذه[2] الحمّى بعض[3] أمراض الدم وكان مزاج العليل مع ذلك دمويا[4] وعروقه ممتلئة وبوله أحمر غليظا[5] وطعم فمه حلوا ونومه كثيرا والزمان[6] فصل الربيع علمنا من هذه الدلائل أنّ الحمّى تولّدت عن[7] احتراق الدم فينبغي عند[8] ذلك أن نستعمل[9] ما[10] يلطّف وينضج المادّة من غير إسخان مثل السكنجبين وحسو الشعير المتّخذ مع[11] السكنجبين. ويؤخذ الورد المربّى والبنفسج المربّى فيمرس في ماء الهندباء[12] وهو حارّ ويصفّى ويشرب وتنزل رجلي العليل في ماء حارّ قد طبخ فيه بابونج ونوّار بنفسج. ويستدعى القيء

680

685

---

^{١٤}ماء: بماء I

^١مضروب: مطبوخ B

^٢هذه الحمّى: هذه العلّة أي الحمّى D

^٣بعض: مع(!) O

^٤دمويا: قويا D دميا I

^٥غليظا: غليظ I

^٦والزمان: والزمن I

^٧عن: من DI

^٨عند ذلك: -I

^٩نستعمل: -O تدبر D يعالج IT

^{١٠}ما: بما DIT

^{١١}مع: معه BDO

^{١٢}الهندباء..حارّ: -T

عند¹ ابتـداء النوائب وعند حـدوث البـرد ويمصّ² مـاء³ الرمّانين ويمزج الماء بالسكنجبين ويلطّف الغذاء.

فإذا نضجت المادّة بادرنا بإخـراج الدم بالفـصـد من الباسليق أو من الأكحل ليسـتفرغ غليظ الدم⁴ ومحترقه وأحدرنا بعد ذلك الطبيعة بالمطبوخات التي ترقّق⁵ الدم وتزيل حـدّته وتكسـر وهجـه. فإذا جاوزت⁶ هذه الحـمّى عشـرين يومـا⁷ ألزمنا⁸ العليل الصـوم في كلّ يوم نوبة وتخـفـيف⁹ طعامه في غير أيام النوائب.

فإن تقدّم هذه الحمّى بعض الأمراض البلغمانية وكان العليل شيخـا مرطوبا ومزاجه باردا ونبضه بطيئا وبوله نيئا غليظا أبيض¹⁰ وعطشـه قليلا وكان الزمـان شـتـاء وطبـيـعـة الهـواء الحـاضـر¹¹ باردة رطبـة علمنا من هذه¹² الدلائل أنّ

---

¹ عند: في IT

² ويمصّ: ويقتصر على D

³ ماء: -IT

⁴ الدم ومحترقه: المادّة المحترقة I

⁵ ترقّق: توافق I

⁶ جاوزت: جازت B

⁷ يوما: -O

⁸ ألزمنا العليل الصوم: أمرمنا العليل بالصوم B

⁹ وتخفيف: وخفّف DIOT

¹⁰ أبيض: أبيضا IT

¹¹ الحاضر: الباردة T

690

695

الحمّى تولّدت عن تشيّط‮'‬ البلغم واحتراقه فينبغي عند ذلك
أن يسقى العليل في الابتداء من‮'‬ ماء الهندباء وماء
الرازيانج وماء الكرفس من الجميع نصف رطل مغلّى مصفّى
ويمرس فيه ورد‮'‬ مربّى بالعسل‮'‬ وبنفسج‮'‬ مربّى بالعسل
من كلّ واحد وزن عشرة دراهم ويصفّى ويشرب.

فإن تعذّرت الطبيعة أحدرناها بماء‮'‬ اللبلاب مع السكّر أو
بحقنة قوية تحدر المادّة إلى أسفل. ويمرخون أبدانهم بأدهان
حارّة مفتّحة للمسامّ مستجلبة للعرق‮'‬ ويمنعون من الطعام
يوم النوبة إلا أن تكون القوّة قد ضعفت، ويتناولون‮'‬ من
الطعام الشيء اليسير ويستعملون‮'‬ من الشراب ما كان
لطيفا معتدل‮'‬ الحرارة ومن الطير ما كان لحمه ليّنا رخصا.

‮'‬هذه الدلائل: ذلك O

‮'‬تشيّط: -D

‮'‬من: -I

‮'‬ورد مربّى: مربّى ورد D

‮'‬بالعسل: -T

‮'‬وبنفسج مربّى بالعسل: -O ومربّى بنفسج عسلي كذلك D

‮'‬بماء اللبلاب: باللبلاب I

‮'‬للعرق: للعروق IT

‮'‬ويتناولون: ويتناولوا T

‮'‬ويستعملون: ويستعملوا T

‮'‬معتدل الحرارة: معتدلا حرارته D

ويغــذون ١ بماء الحـــمّص بأضــلاع ٢ السلق وأصــوله ٣ 710
ويتّقون ٤ جميع ما يبرد ويرطب ويتناولون ٥ بعقب ٦ طعامهم
الجــوارش الكمّــوني والجــوارش المتّــخذ بالثــلاثة ٧ فلافل
وجـوارش الآنيـسون ولا بأس أن يتـقيّـؤوا ٨ إمّــا ٩ بورق ١٠
الفجل وماء الشبثّ أو ١١ بالسكنجبين العسلي قد أنقع فيه
فجل مقطّع من الليل إلى الصبح، ويتعاهدون ١٢ أخذ ترياق 715
الفاروق ودواء القسط ودواء الراوند ودواء الكبريت وما أشبه
ذلك من المعجونات.

فـإذا جـاوزت العلّة ١٣ ثلاثة أسـابيع يغـذوا ١٤ بالفـراريج

---

١ ويغذون: ويغذوا T

٢ بأضلاع: باصلاح D وأضلاع I

٣ وأصوله: -T

٤ ويتّقون: ويتوقون DI ويسقون O ويتوقوا T

٥ ويتناولون: ويتناولوا T

٦ بعقب: بعد BI

٧ بالثلاثة: بالثلاث IT

٨ يتقيّؤوا: يتنقوا B يترقوا(؟) B² يتقيون IO

٩ إمّا: -IT

١٠ بورق الفجل: بالفجل I

١١ أو: و- IT

١٢ ويتعاهدون: ويتعاهدوا I

١٣ العلّة...والدرّاج: -B

١٤ يغذوا: يغذون DO

والدرّاج، فـإذا جـاوزت الحمّى أربعين يومـا يتناولوا¹ لحم²
الحمـلان الحوليـة ويستـعمـلون³ الأدوية ألتي تفتح السـدد⁴
وتدرّ البول وتقوّي الأحشاء. فهذا تدبير حمّى الربع المتولّدة
عن عـفـونة المرّة⁵ السوداء والمتولّدة عن احـتـراق الأخـلاط
باختصار وايجاز وفيه كفاية.

الباب السادس⁶ في الحمّى النائبة⁷ كلّ يوم
إنّ هذه الحمّى التي تنوب⁸ كلّ يوم إنّما تتولّد عن عفـونة
كيموس البلغم وقد بيّن أفاضل الأطّباء في⁹ موضوعاتهم¹⁰
أنّ كلّ مادّة كـانت¹¹ بلغمـانية أو صفـراوية أو سوداوية إذا¹²

720

725

---

¹يتناولوا: يتناولون BDO

²لحم: لحوم BI الحمام و– DT

³ويستعملون: ويستعملوا T

⁴السدد: ‐BDOT

⁵المرّة السوداء: السوداء BDO السدد T

⁶السادس: الخامس O + من المقالة السابعة B

⁷النائبة: + في T

⁸تنوب: + في T

⁹في: من T

¹⁰موضوعاتهم: موضعهم D

¹¹كانت: ‐T

¹²إذا عفنت: ‐O

عفنت اكتسبت غليانا وفورانا وتولّد عن¹ الغليـان والفوران

730 حرارة² وحمّى. فكذلك البلغم إذا عفن وكان مبثوثا في البدن
وكان داخل العروق والأوراد ولّد حمّى تسمّى باليونانية *
امـفـيـمـارينوس³ أي⁴ الدائمـة التي⁵ لا تنكسـر ولا يـحـدث
معها برد .

وإن كانت عفونة البلغم خارج العروق والأوراد ولّد الحمّى
الدائرة ذات النوائب التي تتـرك وتأخـذ في⁶ كلّ يوم ويكون

735 مقدار مدّة⁷ نوبتـها ثماني عشـر⁸ سـاعـة وسكونها ستّ
سـاعات ويستدلّ على هذه الحمّى بالثلاث⁹ دلائل التي يستدلّ
بهـا على حمّى الغبّ وعلى حـمّى الربع أعني من الأشياء
الطبيعية¹⁰ والأشياء التي ليست بطبيعية¹¹ والأشياء الخارجة

---

¹عن: + دلك I

²حرارة...العروق: -D

³*امفيمارينوس: مقتمارينوس B مقيمارسوس DT اسقمارينوس I

اسفيارينوس O

⁴أي: -BDI

⁵التي: + لا تنفصل و- O

⁶في: -O

⁷مدّة: -DO

⁸ثماني عشر: ثمانية عشر D ثمان عشرة O

⁹بالثلاث: بثلاث B

¹⁰والأشياء...الأشياء الطبيعية: -O

¹¹بطبيعية والأشياء الخارجة: طبيعية الخارجة B

740 من¹ الطبيعة.

فأمّا² الاستدلال عليها من الأشياء³ الطبيعية وهو *
أنّها⁴ أكثر ما تعرض لمن كان مزاجه باردا رطبا وسنّه⁵
شيخا أو صبيا لغلبة البلغم على سنّ المشائخ بالطبع وعلى
سنّ الصبيان بالعرض. فأمّا الاستدلال عليها من الأشياء
745 التي ليست بطبيعية فهو أنّها⁶ أكثر ما تتولّد في زمان⁷
الشتاء وإذا كان مزاج الهواء الحاضر مشاكلا⁸ لطبيعة
الزمان في البرودة والرطوبة ومزاج البلدة كذلك وبخاصّة إذا
كان العليل في حال صحّته مدمنا⁹ على الدعة والسكون كثير
الترفة قليل التعب والنصب. وأمّا الاستدلال عليها من الأشياء
الخارجة من¹⁰ الطبيعة فهو أنّ هذه الحمّى تعرض لأصحابها
750 في الابتداء ببرد¹¹ شديد شبيه بالزمهرير يبرد منه البدن كلّه

---

¹من: عن I

²فأمّا: فإنّما B

³الأشياء الطبيعية: الأشياء الخارجة من الطبيعية T

⁴وهو *أنّها: فهو أنّه B فإنّه D وهو أن IOT

⁵وسنه: وشبه(!) D

⁶أنّها: -T أيضا D أنّ O

⁷زمان: زمن I

⁸مشاكلا: مشاكل I

⁹مدمنا على: قد اعتاد على D

¹⁰من: عن B

¹¹ببرد: برد BDIT

حـتّى يصل ذلك إلى أطراف اليـدين والرجلين ويمكث ذلك
بصاحبه[1] ساعة. فـإذا عفن البلغم وحمي تصاعدت حرارته
رويدا رويدا وزال البرد وكانت الحمّى خفيفة رطبة الحركة إلا
أنّها مـتطاولة مخوفة[2] وهذه الحمّى مقرونة بألم المعدة وذلك
أنّ أكثر تولّد البلغم في أكثر الحالات إنّما يكون في فم المعدة
ولذلك يتقيّؤون قيئًا بلغمانيا ويعرض لهم الغثي[3] وتتهبّج[4]
وجـوهـهم وتصـيـر ألوانهم رصاصية مـائلة إلى البيـاض
والكمودة[5] وتكون أفواهـهم رطبة وأكثر ذلك لا يعطشون.

وإنّما يصل[6] المتطبّب إلى كيـفـيـة عـلاج هذه الحمّى
وصـورتهـا[7] من طبيـعـة البلغم وذلك أنّ من البلغم البارد[8]
الرطب وعلى[9] الحـقـيـقـة وهو النوع[10] الطبـيـعي المتولّد عن[11]

---

[1] بصاحبه: في صاحبه D

[2] مخوفة: محرقة B

[3] الغثي: الغشى DIT القيء O

[4] وتتهبّج: وتهبج B وتتهيّج DO وتهيج I

[5] والكمودة: والكمود OT

[6] يصل: يصير I

[7] وصورتها: وصورته B وسورته IT وحدوثه D

[8] البارد الرطب: بارد رطب B ما هو بارد رطب O

[9] وعلى: على BDIT

[10] النوع: اللون O

[11] عن صفو الدم: عن غلبة البرد على صفو الدم T

صفـو الدم ومـائيتـه¹، ومنه مـا هو² أبرد وأغلظ وأقلّ رطوبة
مـثل³ البلغم الحـامض المتـولّد عن⁴ غلبـة البـرد على صفـو
الدم ومـائيته، ومنه⁵ مـا هو أسـخن وأجفّ مـثل⁶ البلغم المالح
المتولّد عن⁷ غلبة الحرارة على صفو الدم ومائيته.⁸

فإذا وجد العليل مع الحمّى عطشا وجفاف الفم تبيّن⁹ لنا
أنّ تولّد الحمّى من بلغم¹⁰ مـالح وأمـرنا عند ذلك أن يعطى
العليل السكنجبين السكّري والماء الحارّ على الريق فإذا جاء
وقت النوبة وحدث البرد أنزلوا أرجلهم في ماء قد طبخ فيه
بابونج وشبثّ ونوّار بنفسج ويدلك¹¹ تحت القدمين بملح ودهن
بنفسج.

فـإذا جـاء القيء طوعـا في ابتـداء المرض دلّ على لطافة

---

¹ومائيته: ومباينته B

²هو: + أسخن وأجفّ O

³مثل: وهو I

⁴عن..ومائيته: -B

⁵ومنه..ومائيته: -I

⁶مثل: من O

⁷عن: من O

⁸ومائيته: ومباينته B

⁹تبيّن لنا: بيّنا BT تبيّن O تبيّنا I

¹⁰بلغم: + لزج I

¹¹ويدلك: ويدهن B

الفضل وخفّته وسرعة حركته، فإن لم يأت' القيء طوعا
فلا' تستجلبه كرها' لأنّ امتناع القيء في ابتداء' المرض
دالّ' على أنّ' الفضل غليظ جامد' ممتنع الذوبان بطيء
الحركة، ويأكل' العليل وردا' مربّى سكّريا ويشرب عليه
ماء حارًا'' لأنّ الماء الحارّ محمود في هذه الحمّى'' جدّا''
لأنّه يذيب المادّة ويلطّفها ويحلّلها. ثمّ يتناول بعد الورد المربّى
بساعة حسو الشعير مع السكنجبين السكّري.''

فإن كانت الطبيعة مجيبة وإلا فيعطون من ماء اللبلاب إلى
نصف رطل مع أوقية سكّر سليماني أو يحلّ فيه ترنجبين

775

780

' يأت: يأتي O

' فلا: -DO

' كرها: طوعا D

' ابتداء: أوّل O أوائل T

' دالّ: دلّ I

' أنّ: -D

' جامد: خامل B

' ويأكل: ويأخذ D

' وردا مربّى سكّريا: ورد مربّى سكّري DOT وردا مربّى سكّري I

'' حارًا: حارّ BDOT

'' الحمّى: العلّة أي الحمّى D

'' جدّا: -I

'' السكّري: عسلي O

خراساني وورد مربّى¹ من كلّ واحد أوقية ويصفّى ويشرب.
فإن أجابت الطبيعة بذلك وإلا فتتّخذ لهم حقنة² لطيفة أو
فتل³ مسهلة.⁴

785

فإن ذكر⁵ العليل أنّه يحسّ نفخا وقراقرا في أمعائه⁶ أو
شكى⁷ غثيانا⁸ وتقلّبا⁹ في معدته علمنا عند ذلك أنّ المادّة
قد ذابت وسالت وطلبت الخروج. أمّا بالإسهال إن كان يجد¹⁰
نفخا وقراقرا فيجب أن تعين¹¹ الطبيعة على إخراج المادّة
بلطافة ورفق مثل¹² أن يسقى العليل مطبوخا¹³ لطيفا مأمونا

790

أو حبوبا على مثل ذلك أو يسقى أقراص الورد المسهلة وما

---

¹ مربّى: O-

² حقنة: + ليّنة D

³ فتل: شربة O

⁴ مسهلة: B¹ مستعملة B سهلة I

⁵ ذكر العليل: كان العليل ذكر T

⁶ أمعائه: أمعائها I

⁷ شكى: اشتكى B

⁸ غثيانا: غليانا I

⁹ وتقلّبا: وثقلا B

¹⁰ يجد: D-

¹¹ تعين: يلين(!) T

¹² مثل: بمثل T على O

¹³ مطبوخا لطيفا مأمونا أو حبوبا: مطبوخ لطيف مأمون أو حبوب I

أشبه ذلك. فإن شكى غثيانا وتقلّبا[1] في معدته أمرنا العليل
عند[2] ابتداء البرد من[3] كلّ نوبة أن يشرب السكنجبين
السكّري وماء[4] الشبثّ مطبوخا ويستجلب القيء من غير
عنف على المعدة.

795

فإن لم يكن في قوّة البدن[5] احتمال الأدوية المسهلة
فيحتال في تدبيرهم بتلطيف المادّة وتنقيتها من غير عنف على
الطبيعة، ويكون ذلك على حسب طبيعة المادّة والغالب[6] عليها
وطبيعة العضو الذي المادّة مائلة إليه. فإن كانت المادّة بلغما
مالحا وكانت مائلة نحو الكبد سقيناه[7] من الأدوية ما كان

800

مخصوصا بتنظيف[8] الكبد[9] وتلطيف المادّة وإخراجها[10]
بالبول مثل أقراص الطباشير أو أقراص الكافور أو أقراص

---

[1] وتقلّبا: وثقلا B

[2] عند ابتداء: عند ذلك في ابتداء T

[3] من: في B من كلّ نوبة: قبل نوبة O

[4] وماء الشبثّ مطبوخا: وماء شبثّ مطبوخ B وماء شبثّ مطبوخا D وماء
الشبثّ مطبوخ I

[5] البدن: العليل I

[6] والغالب: والغلبة T

[7] سقيناه: اسقيناه IT

[8] بتنظيف: بتلطيف I

[9] الكبد: البدن D

[10] وإخراجها: ويخرجها BIT

الصندل مع السكنجبين السكّري. فإن كان البلغم حامضا[1]
فيسقى أقراص الورد أو أقراص البرباريس[2] أو أقراص
الآنيسون مع[3] ماء الهندباء وماء الرازيانج وماء الكرفس
من[4] جميعها نصف رطل مع أوقية شراب سكنجبين عسلي،
وقرصة[5] من أحد[6] هذه الأقراص التي[7] ذكرنا ويلزم مثل
هذا التدبير أسبوعا.[8]

فإن طالت الحمى ولم تذهب بمثل هذا التدبير فيعطون
مطبوخ الأصول على ما ذكرنا[9] في المقالة الخامسة[10] من
هذا الكتاب أو[11] شراب الإذخر أو شراب الأفسنتين، فإن
كانت المادّة مائلة نحو المعدة وكان البلغم حامضا فينبغي أن
نعالج في ابتداء المرض بشراب العسل وماء حارّ أو شراب

---

[1] حامضا: مالحا I

[2] البرباريس: الرنباس(!) T

[3] مع: في I

[4] من جميعها: جميعا B

[5] وقرصة: أو قرص B

[6] أحد: احدي O

[7] التي: الذي BO

[8] أسبوعا: أسبوع I

[9] ذكرنا: ذكرناه B ذكرته T

[10] الخامسة: + من هذا الكتاب B

[11] أو: -O

سكنجبين عسلي وماء حارّ ويغذوا ` بحسو الشعير
المطبوخ ` مع قشور أصول الرازيانج وأصول الكرفس ويلقى
عليه بعد تصفيته سكنجبين عسلي. `

ويسقون في وقت يعرض لهم البرد عند ابتداء نوبة الحمّى
ماء الشبثّ وشراب سكنجبين عسلي مع فجل مقطّع `
ويستدعوا ` القيء وتنزل ` أرجلهم في ماء قد طبخ فيه
بابونج وشبثّ وإكليل الملك ونمام وقيصوم. فإن جاءهم القيء
طوعا فلا يمتنعون منه وبخاصّة في ابتداء المرض ويعطى `
الورد المربّى العسلي بالماء الحارّ. فإذا نضج الفضل فيسقى
عند ذلك نقيع الصبر أو نقيع الإيارج أو مطبوخ الأفسنتين أو
حبّ المصتكى والصبر.

فإن كانت قوّة ` العليل تضعف عن احتمال ما وصفنا
فيعطى ` أقراص الغافت أو أقراص الأفسنتين أو أقراص

` ويغذوا: ويغذون BD

` المطبوخ: -I

` عسلي: -I

` مقطّع: مقطوع I

` ويستدعوا: ويستدعون B

` وتنزل: وتترك T وتنزل...في ابتداء المرض: -D

` ويعطى: ويعطوا DT + قليل D

` قوّة: -I

` فيعطى: فيسقى O

الراوند مع مياه البقول وشراب سكنجبين عسلي ويستدعوا¹
القيء عند ابتـداء النوبة² ويمتنعوا³ من الغـذاء إلى أن
تنقضي سورة الحمّى ولا يقصدوا⁴ من التدبير⁵ ألطفه⁶
لأنّ هذه الحمّى فيها⁷ طول مدّة وبعد انحلال.

830

فـإذا قـصـدوا من التـدبيـر ألطفه مع طول مـدّة المرض
حارت⁸ القوّة وضـعفت، وإذا ظهر لنا دلائل النضج في البول
فـينبغي أن نكمّد المعدة ونمرخها⁹ بأشياء مقـوّية مـزيلة
للفضـول عنها مثل دهن النـاردين أو دهن المصطكى أو دهن
الأفسنتين أو دهن الشبثّ وما أشبه ذلك من الأدهان وتكمّد¹⁰

835

بماء قد طبخ فيه بابونج وسنبل ومصطكى وأفسنتين وما أشبه
ذلك. وتضمّد بضمادات حارّة معتدلة عطرية ويمزجوا¹¹ الماء

---

¹ويستدعوا: ويستدعون BD

²النوبة: العلّة O

³ويمتنعوا: ويمنعون B ويمتنعون D

⁴يقصدوا: يقصدون BDIO

⁵التدبير: + إلا BO

⁶ألطفه: ألطيف D

⁷فيها طول: أطول D

⁸حارت: خارت BD

⁹ونمرخها: وتمزجها D

¹⁰وتكمّد: ونكمّدها I

¹¹ويمزجوا: ويمزجون DI ويخرج (!) O

بالشراب¹ الرفيـع أو شـراب العـسـل المطبـوخ بـالأفـاويه
ويسـقوا² من الأدوية النافعـة لمن³ به فـسـاد المعدة لأنّ هذه
الحمّى مخصوصة بألم المعدة كما بيّنّا⁴ وشرحنا .

840

---

¹بالشراب الرفيع: بالشراب الرقيـق D بشراب النعنع T

²ويسقوا : ويسقون BDO

³لمن به: المرية B لمن كان به O

⁴بيّنّا: ذكرنا B

TRANSLATION

In the name of God, the Merciful, the Compassionate

The seventh treatise from the book *Provisions for the Traveller*

In the previous treatises we have with God's help - may He be praised - dealt with the [different] diseases which occur in the internal organs. We have elucidated the [different kinds of] treatment for those diseases in the best possible and most direct way, [while referring to] their most immediate source. In this seventh treatise which will be the seal of this eminent book, I will mention those external diseases that can be noticed by the senses and those that are accompanied by pain that is felt by the internal organs. I will also mention the different ways of treating these diseases according to the methods of medicine and rules of our profession.

I will begin with an exposition of fever, because it is, as Galen stated, the most dangerous disease, the messenger of death, and the most frequent cause of the end of life[1], because it encompasses both the external and internal [parts of] the body. Moreover, it is harmful for the pneumata, the psychical faculties, and the natural activities [of the body]. I will start my discussion with ephemeral fever which arises in the pneumata, for this fever often has a most immediate cause which in its turn causes

---

[1] "End of life" (*ajal*). For this concept and its role in Islamic theology see now B. Abrahamow, "The appointed time of death (*aǧal*) according to 'Abd al-Ǧabbār."

other fevers to arise. But other fevers do not cause this fever in any way. Then I will mention [other] diseases in the same order as in the beginning of the book.

Chapter one: On ephemeral fever

Ephemeral fever arises from excessive heat which heats the pneumata, but not any material part [of the body]; nor does it arise from putrefaction. It therefore does not last longer than one day. By pneumata I understand the animal pneuma which is the source of life and the matter of the innate heat, the psychical pneuma which is the source of sensation and movement, and the natural pneuma which is the source of the four natural faculties, namely, the attractive faculty, the retentive faculty, the digesting faculty, and the excretory faculty.

This fever can be divided into two [different] kinds: One is the disease itself, the other is accidental to the disease and follows the preceding disease. The kind of fever which is the disease itself has three [possible] causes: 1. External, with respect to the outside of the body, such as the heat of the sun in the summer, a hot sandstorm (*simoon*), severe cold, and bathing in waters which have the power to dry the outside of the bodies and to thicken them (i.e. to obstruct the pores of the skin), such as water containing natron, alum, and sulphur. 2. An excess of bodily movement, such as strain, exertion, continuous walking and the like, and excessive emotions, such as great anger, continuous worrying, and other psychical afflictions. 3. Continuous consumption of

hot foods and of drinks which heat the blood, and the like. As
for the ephemeral fever which is accidental following a preceding
disease, it is like the fever following inflammations of the groin,
armpit, neck, and the like. For if the blood which is present in
the inflammation stays in it and is not quickly dissolved, it becomes
hot, putrefies, and heats the animal pneuma. This heat then reaches
the heart because of the connection between the arteries and the
heart, and the result of this is ephemeral fever. These are all the
causes of ephemeral fever.

Now I will discuss specifically every single cause [of this
fever] and its symptoms, and then I will in an orderly and concise
way deal with the treatment useful for those suffering from this
fever. The symptoms for ephemeral fever caused by the heat of
the sun are that the heads of those suffering from it are warm,
and that they are warmer than the rest of their body. For the
glare of the sun reaches their brain, so that they often suffer
from headache and their faces become red and are often affected
by a hot rheum which burns their noses.

As for the fever caused by the burning heat of a hot sandstorm,
the bodies of those suffering from it are warmer than their heads.
The outside of their bodies is inflamed and dry since the heat of
the sandstorm dries the moisture of their bodies.

As for the fever caused by cold and severe frost, its symptoms
are amongst others that the complexion of those suffering from
it changes; it loses its blood-like freshness and beauty, but assumes
the colour and paleness of dust. The outside of their bodies
becomes cold, dry and arid; in addition to cold they feel heaviness

in their heads.

As for those suffering from this fever because they bathed in astringent drying waters, their skins are more dry and arid than the skins of those suffering from this fever because of cold and severe frost. Their skins are in fact so dry that if you touch them with your hand it is as if they were macerated for a while in an infusion of gallnuts and pomegranate peels. And if you leave your hand for some time on a certain place of their body until their skin becomes warm because of the heat of your hand, that part of their body will become loose [again] after it had become congested because their skin had become thick and firm, because of the hot natural evaporations [of the body].[2]

As for ephemeral fever arising from hot foods and drinks, this [kind of] food inflames the blood and natural pneuma by its heat; for the natural pneuma is located in the liver and is transported by the blood. Then the heat reaches the heart and spreads through the whole body. Therefore the urine of those suffering from this kind of ephemeral fever is redder than that of [those suffering from] other types of this fever, because the urine is the wateriness the blood and the place where the [other] humours flow to. [Since this fever comes from the liver] those that suffer from it find, when this fever subsides, that their liver is hot.

As for ephemeral fever arising from bodily exertion, the bodies of those suffering from it become thin, arid and dry; they feel a severe weakness and constant heavy pain in their joints. When

---

[2] These evaporations had been prevented from leaving the body, thus causing the heat to collect in it; cf. Paul of Aegina, *op. cit.*, Bk. 2, ch. 17; al-Mājūsī, *op. cit.*, Bk. 1, discourse 8, ch. 3, p. 348.

their fever subsides, their perspiration is unlike that [occurring] in the other kinds of ephemeral fever. For when the impression of this fever diminishes and subsides, a moisture is dissolved from the body [of the patient] that is similar to the moisture of the bodies [of those] that come out of a bath. Some patients transpire profusely, but if there is neither moisture nor perspiration there is necessarily much vapour that arises from the depth of the body.

As for ephemeral fever arising from anger and fury, its symptoms are a red complexion, bulging and quickly moving eyes, dry eyelids, and a strong and powerful pulse of those suffering from it. Sometimes their complexion turns pale and a tremor befalls them; this happens when the anger and fury is mixed with fear.

As for ephemeral fever arising from grief or worry, the eyes of those suffering from it are hollow and motionless; their faces lose their freshness and their complexion becomes ugly; their bodies become thin; their pulses weak; their urine red. These symptoms are common to those who are worried or grieved in any way, but this [kind of fever] is best recognised from the condition of the eyes, for the eyes of him who grieves or is worried are dry. [The symptom of] hollow eyes is common to all those who suffer from these afflictions, i.e. worry, grief, and insomnia. All of them have in common that their urine is yellowish, while he who suffers from this fever because of grief, has a body containing heat that is rather intense [in quality] than large in quantity. When the physician knows the cause of the fever that lasts for one day - for this has become clear to him from the signs and symptoms that I have mentioned - he should let those who suffer from it take a bath quickly.

If the fever has been caused by the heat of the sun or by a sandstorm, those [who suffer from it] should enter the bathhouse when the fever subsides and its severity is over; they should, however, not stay in it for a long time. One should spread before them aromatic plants which alleviate the vapour [arising from their bodies], such as roses, violets, Egyptian willow, and leaves of fleawort. Their noses should be moistened all the time with oil of violets, oil of nenuphar; their temples should be rubbed with oil of roses mixed with vinegar. Once the fever has subsided one should pour over their heads water in which violet blossoms and camomile have been cooked, but only if they do neither have a cold nor a headache. One should also beware of doing this when their heads contain any amount [of phlegm], for then they should only bend themselves over their vapours [in order to inhale them]. One should let them drink juice of the two kinds of pomegranates[3] with crystalline sugar, and they should take medicinal drinks prepared from rose-water syrup, violets, roses, and plums. They should be fed with bread pulp that has been washed with crystalline sugar; one may also feed them with gourd, purslane, kernels of cucumber, and core of lettuce, and one should let them suck pomegranate. When the heat [of the sun] has subsided, they should be fed with [the meat of] francolins

---

[3] The sweet and acidulous varieties of the cultivated pomegranate; see Latham-Isaacs, *K. al-ḥummāyāt*, p. 88, n. 72.

and chickens with juice of the two kinds of pomegranates or juice of unripe, sour grapes.

When the fever has been caused by cold and severe frost, they who suffer from it should, once the superfluous humour has matured and the fever has been overcome, put their feet into water in which camomile, marjoram, aneth, and thyme have been cooked; they should also bend themselves over its vapours [and inhale them]. They should take a bath with sweet waters, but spend more time in the bathhouse itself than in the bath, for the air of the bathhouse makes their bodies transpire, dissolves their moisture, and opens their pores. If those suffering from this fever have a catarrh caused by the cold, they should only take a bath when this superfluous humour has matured and then been dissolved. They should inhale pure vapours, such as [those of] marjoram, jasmine, gillyflower, and the like. They should cover themselves with clothes, while close to them coalfires should be kindled, so that the cold air will not reach them. Their heads should be anointed with oils of a moderate heat, such as oil of camomile, aneth, gillyflower, lily, and the like.

If this fever has been caused by washing with astringent drying waters, those suffering from it should only take a bath when the fever has subsided in severity and has been overcome and after they have put their feet into water in which camomile, aneth, marjoram, and the like have been cooked. They should also bend themselves over the vapour of the water [in order to inhale it]. When they take a bath, they should rub their bodies softly and pour sweet lukewarm water over them, for this softens their skins and opens their pores. But they should beware of anointing themselves when they take a bath, for this closes the pores of their bodies and blocks their inner vapours. Moderate physical exercise is one of the best means to treat this fever, because it loosens the bodies, opens their pores, and dissolves the vapours blocked in them. In short, they who suffer from this fever should beware of everything that cools the skin, contracts it, and closes its pores; they should be fed with that which is quickly digested and drink sugar mixed with water.

If this fever is caused by hot foods, the patient should be given to drink oxymel prepared with sugar or juice of the two kinds of pomegranates mixed with rose-water syrup or with crystalline sugar. When the fever has subsided one should administer him *tabāshīr* pastilles[4] or camphor pastilles with a drink made of violets or roses. To his liver one should apply a warm pack with duck-weed or purslane and mucilage of fleawort seed and gourd peels, or with sandalwood, barley meal and some camphor kneaded with juice of roses. For food the patient should take purslane, endive, orache, and gourd; when he is thirsty he should drink water mixed with juice of fleawort seed or of the two kinds of pomegranates.

When this fever is caused by physical exertion, those who

---

[4] *Ṭabāshīr*: cf. Levey, *The medical formulary or Aqrābādhīn of al-Kindī*, p. 300, no. 186: "It is a kind of 'lime' as a concretion in the knots of a particular species of bamboo. It is 'chalk' in Iran and Iraq today. The word is Pers. but may have come from Sans. *twak-kshīrā*, indicating the *Bambusa arundinacea Schreb.*" Cf. Said, *al-Bīrunī's Book on Pharmacy*, p. 218, n.1: "*Ṭabāshīr* denotes the young shoots, seeds and siliceous concretion of Bambusa arundinecea Retz. (family, Graminae).

suffer from it should be required to look for calm and rest; their bodies should be rubbed softly with oil of violets, roses or nenuphar. They should enter a bathhouse with moderately heated air and water, but they should not take a bath for a long time. When they come out of the sweet [moderately] hot water, their bodies should be rubbed with oil of violets or roses; they should be administered juice of the two kinds of pomegranates and violets, or juice of plums, or juice of rose-water syrup. They should be fed with foods that moisten their bodies, such as [the meat of] chickens and of goats, freshwater fish, and the like.

When this fever is caused by excessive emotions, the cause which harms and troubles the soul should be opposed by means which (are opposite and) expel it. Anger, grief, and fury, for instance, should be opposed by words and deeds that appease and please the soul. For they who suffer from it can engage in different kinds of amusement which provide joy and comfort, or look at those things which give relief to the soul, such as green aromatic plants and pleasant faces. In addition to the healing of the soul by that which we mentioned, one should in the case of these patients require from them to cure their bodies by means of that which moistens them and takes away the dryness affecting them. They should, for instance, take a sweet water bath in a bathhouse with moderate [hot] air, and rub their bodies when leaving the lukewarm water with oil of violets or oil of nenuphar, but they should not massage their bodies too much, for this increases their dryness and aridness. Therefore one should forbid them to have sexual intercourse, and to move [too much], and

let them feed themselves with barley broth, gourd, purslane, and
wild-amaranth. When the fever has subsided, they should be fed
with the meat of francolin, chickens and goats. They should take
drinks of a balanced temperament, inhale sandalwood, camphor,
roses, violets, and myrtle, and suck juice of the two kinds of
pomegranates and winter grapes. One should administer them
water-melon juice with crystalline sugar. In short, they should
avoid those things that dry [their bodies], and take those which
moisten [them]. These means should be administered in their
case according to the strength of the patient, his age, natural
temperament and habit, and according to the time of the year,
country, and other similar things.

If this fever occurs to someone because of an inflammation
of the groin, it is [first of all] necessary to treat the inflammation
and to dissolve it, and to cure at the same time the putrefaction
which caused the inflammation. Then he gets a treatment similar
to that mentioned by us above. This is what we wanted to say
about the symptoms of ephemeral fever and its treatment in a
concise way.

Chapter two: On ardent fever

Ardent fever, called *kausos* in Greek, is a fever accompanied by
intense continuous thirst and continuous heat which is harmful
and upsetting for [human] nature, and which incites it to combat
the disease and to confront it from its [very] beginning. [It is so
harmful for human nature] because of the sharpness and pungency

of that element which causes this fever, namely, the sharp, fiery, yellow bile that has collected in the cavities of the veins that are adjacent to the heart, especially those of the cardia of the stomach, of the concave part of the liver, and of the cavity of the lung.

The symptoms belonging to this fever are, [as we stated above], continuous heat and continuous, unremitting thirst. The heat in the case of ardent fever is continuous because of the bilious humour from which it originates inside the veins; the fever becomes solid and continuous because most of the bilious humour which causes it is in the veins adjacent to the heart. And since the bilious humour which causes this fever can, as we explained, especially be found in the veins of the cardia of the stomach and the concave part of the liver, the thirst becomes intense, continuous, and unremitting.

There are two kinds of ardent fever; one authentic and severe, and the other false and light. The authentic and severe one originates from yellow bile pure in sharpness and pungency; it mostly occurs in juveniles and young men, and in those whose temperament is by nature hot and sharp, especially during the summer, because the summertime strengthens this fever and increases it by nature. The light false kind arises from yellow bile mixed with sweet moisture or sweet vapour. Since this fever is very dangerous and frightening, the physician should proceed in it very carefully from the beginning; he should observe the four phases of a disease, namely, beginning, progress, crisis and abatement, and apply in every phase that which is necessary.

When the physician sees in the beginning of the disease that the nature [of the patient] is in need of that which moves the superfluities and evacuates them, he should administer him juice of tamarind, plums, and jujube with the core of reedy Indian laburnum, manna from Khurāsān, preserved violets, a drink made of plums, and the like. In case the physician was unable to stimulate the nature [of the patient] in the beginning of the disease because of an obstacle preventing him from doing so, such as weakness of strength [of the patient] who would not be able to bear an evacuation, or unripeness and crudeness of the superfluity, he should be extremely careful not to do so when the disease is progressing, for if he did so, the nature [of the patient] would become confused regarding its healing activity, and because of this confusion it would abandon managing [the process of] the disease completely. But if [for this reason] the physician has been unable to stimulate the nature [of the patient] in the beginning of the disease, he should assist his nature to regain its power by means of food that is digested quickly and that is commendable for its substance, such as broth of fortified barley or bread pulp that has been washed several times with cold water.

Galen has mentioned in his work *De crisibus* how a physician should feed his patients in the case of acute diseases: There are three criteria which the physician should consider when determining the diet of the patient: 1. The degree of strength [which the patient has] against a disease; 2. The duration of a disease; 3. The quality of a disease. The degree of strength against a disease is amongst those things which should be kept high, since it fights the disease. The physician should therefore provide the patient with much food without paying attention to the time [of the year], when we are afraid that his strength will decline. The duration of a disease should be considered for determining the quality of the food in relation to the nearness and remoteness of the crisis of the disease. For if the crisis is nearby, extremely fine food should be used until the crisis has [actually] arrived, in which case the patient should not be fed at all. If the crisis is far away one should feed [the patient] gradually, little by little until the disease reaches its crisis. [The physician should consider] the quality of the disease, because all those suffering from fever, for instance, need a moist regimen, and if the fever is accompanied by loss of weight, the need for food is so great that sometimes we even feed [the patient] when he [actually] has fever.

If a fever is accompanied by superfluities in the body, one should beware of giving much food [to the patient]; one should in fact only feed him in the intervals between the bouts of fever, but not in the time that it actually occurs. And if there are no intervals between the bouts of the fever in which it subsides, one should feed the patient [only] when the fever subsides. If, however, the fever does not subside and we have to feed the patient, we chose the time when the patient used to eat when he was healthy; especially good is that time of the day when it is cool and moist, such as the morning, for then his nature is [very] active, the air is mild, and the fever has subsided because the cold of the morning resisted and suppressed its heat and acuteness. This is the end of what the wise physician and philosopher Galen has said in his very words about the best way to feed a patient suffering from an [acute] disease. We have quoted it because of its enormous usefulness and great benefit for [our discussion of] this subject in this book.

When the ardent fever is high and severe from its beginning until its end, we should confine [the patient] to a mild regimen of, for instance, barley broth, washed bread pulp, to which pulverised crystalline sugar has been added. From time to time he should be administered those ingredients that abate the heat of the stomach, such as seedless pomegranate [juice] that should be sucked, winter grapes, and pulp of the green and raw watermelon. One should extract mucilage of fleawort seed in watermelon juice and administer it to the patient. One should also give him a drink made of violets, plums or fleawort seed or exquisite rose-water syrup. In the evening one should give him two *dirhams*[5] of fleawort seed washed in cold water and one *dirham* of purslane seed or five ounces[6] of Armenian earth with sweet pomegranate juice and ten *dirhams* of pulverised Sulaymān sugar[7] or a drink made of violets.

When the patient has been given in the morning juice of barley with juice of sweet pomegranate or a drink made of violets and he needs food, for this does not support him, one should

---

[5] One standard *dirham* is 3,125 grams; see Hinz, *Islamische Masse und Gewichte*, pp. 3-4.

[6] For the varying weights of the ounce see Hinz, *op. cit.*, pp. 34-35; in Egypt it was 37,5 grams.

[7] Freytag, *Lexicon*, vol. 2, p. 334, remarks about this kind of sugar that it is "saccharum purissimum" (very pure sugar).

give him bread crumbs washed with sweet pomegranate juice, or gruel of parched barley washed several times with cold water and crystalline sugar. This should only be done when the fever has abated somewhat, but when it is vehement one should beware of doing so unless it is necessary.

In case the nature [of the patient] suffers from constipation, we soften it before the paroxysm of the disease. We do so by taking juice of gourd in which ten *dirhams* of manna from Khurāsān and ten *dirhams* of preserved violets have been macerated, by broiling this in exactly half a *ratl*[8] of barley dough, by straining this and adding one ounce of pure plum juice to the strained substance, and by administering this to the patient. If you want to make it slightly stronger, you should add five *dirhams* of the core of purified Indian laburnum without its cane and seed. One may also administer to him an infusion of black plums and tamarind with a drink made of violets and manna from Khurāsān.

If the nature [of the patient] responds to this, [it is fine], but if not, one should apply a suppository prepared from violet leaves and natron, half a *mithqāl*[9] of each; half a *dirham* of scammony and one *mithqāl* of lycium. Pulverise these ingredients, dissolve the lycium in hot water, knead the other ingredients with it and make suppositories like acorns from it. Smear oil of violets on these suppositories and apply them.

---

[8] For the varying weights of the *ratl* see Hinz, *op. cit.*, pp. 3, 28-33. In Fatimid Egypt it was 437,2 grams.

[9] One *mithqāl* is 4,464 grams; see Hinz, *op. cit.*, p. 4.

If the nature [of the patient] responds to this, [it is fine], but if not, one should prepare for him a clyster with bramble juice, beet juice and bran extract, two ounces of each; a drink made of violets, plums, and oil of violets, one ounce of each; and one *dirham* of pounded natron. This should be mixed, made lukewarm and applied. The stomach should be moistened and its heat abated with mucilage of fleawort seed and pomegranate juice or with water-melon juice. The stomach should be empty of food during the paroxysm of the disease unless it is necessary [to take something], as, for instance, in the case when there is a danger that the strength [of the patient] is weakened during the struggle between his nature and the disease. For then you should strengthen it with some barley extract or boiled bread crumbs, but only so much as is enough to maintain his strength.

If the patient gets a headache, one should take oil of roses, mix it with wine vinegar or purslane juice or juice of gourd peels and rub it on his forehead and temples. One should also take oil of violets and nenuphar and apply it as an errhine. One should mix this, when it is cold, with rose-water in mucilage of fleawort seed and put it on the forehead and temples. The feet and legs should be put in warm sweet water and rubbed with oil of violets, while the legs should be bandaged. On the forehead and temples should be placed a pack prepared from rubbed sandalwood, barley meal and rose leaves, and kneaded with rose-water or duck-weed juice, juice of gourd peels, purslane juice or mucilage of fleawort seed.

When the patient suffers from insomnia (and sleepnessness),

one should add to the pack lettuce seed and poppy seed which should be kneaded with lettuce juice. The patient should have oil of nenuphar and oil of violets injected into his nose. When his mouth becomes dry and his tongue rough, he should chew mucilage of fleawort seed and quince seed to which some crystalline sugar and oil of violets have been added. When his tongue is black, the mucilages should be mixed with rose-water and oil of roses, and the tongue should be rubbed with this. He may also hold sweet pomegranate juice mixed with oil of roses in his mouth.

If palpitation occurs to the patient, he should be administered mucilage of fleawort seed extracted in cucumber juice with a drink of rose-water syrup, or pomegranate or unripe, sour grapes, or juice of cedrat pulp. One should apply to his stomach a pack prepared from the two kinds of sandalwood and barley meal kneaded with rose-water. One may also take duck-weed, purslane, mucilage of fleawort seed, gourd peels, mix this with rose-water or oil of roses and apply it to the stomach or liver when they are free of food. One should administer to him gruel of parched barley that has been washed several times after one has added crystalline sugar, or rose-water syrup or sweet pomegranate. One should feed him with gourd prepared with juice of unripe, sour grapes, cedrat pulp and purslane stalks. One should also feed him with husked lentils boiled with gourd, crystalline sugar, juice of unripe, sour grapes or some vinegar. One should spread myrtle, Egyptian willow and roses in front of the patient, and sprinkle these plants[10] with water from time to time.

This fever is often accompanied by phrenitis,[11] dry cough, fainting, or jaundice. When this happens one should treat it with the wholesome regimen that we have described in a special chapter of this book.[12]

Chapter three: On tertian fever

Tertian fever is called "tritaios" in Greek which is "muthallatha" in Arabic. This fever originates from yellow bile when it is changed and putrefied. When the putrefaction occurs outside the veins and arteries, it causes intermittent tertian fever which attacks and abates, and is accompanied by cold, shuddering and tremor. And when the putrefaction is inside the veins it causes either continuous tertian fever or the fever [called] "kausos", i.e. burning fever.

If someone asks about the similarity and difference between ardent fever and continuous tertian fever, we answer him that they are similar in so far as both originate from the hot yellow humour, both occur inside the veins and arteries, and both are continuous. They differ in so far as the bilious humour which causes the fever collects in different places. In the case of ardent fever the inflammation occurs in the veins adjacent to the heart

[10] The Hebrew versions of MSS Munich 19 and Parma 1044 have "'ashakhim" (testicles) for "rayḥān" (plants).

[11] The Arabic "birsām" can mean either "pleurisy" or "phrenitis", a now outdated term, at one time denoting either "inflammation of the brain" or "delirium" (See Latham-Isaacs, *op. cit.*, p. 102, n. 103).

[12] Phrenitis is discussed in Bk. 1, ch. 18; cough in Bk. 3, ch. 6, fainting in Bk. 3, ch. 14, and jaundice in Bk. 5, ch. 10.

and especially the veins of the cardia of the stomach, liver and lungs, rather than the veins of the rest of the body, because the [putrefying] matter is more extensive over there, as we explained above. But in the case of continuous tertian fever the inflammation occurring in all the veins of the body is like that occurring in the vessels adjacent to the heart.

There are three things indicating tertian fever, namely, natural, unnatural and extra-natural. It is indicated by natural things in so far as it mostly originates in someone whose temperament is hot and dry and who is between twenty-two and thirty-five years old, especially when his body is lean and its pores open. It is indicated by unnatural things in so far as it mostly originates during the summer, especially when the current weather is hot and dry and the temperament of the country is similar, and when the patient's occupation when he is healthy involves exertion, strain and fatigue. It is indicated by extra-natural things, namely, the symptoms originating from the nature of the element that causes the fever. These symptoms are afflictions for the patient and signs and indications for the physician. For since this fever originates from the hot bilious element that is adjacent to the sensory organs, it must be preceded by heavy shuddering and [the sensation of] pricking like that caused by needles and thorns. For the bilious sharp humour, when it passes and flows through the sensory organs which are not used to it, causes a biting sensation because of its sharpness. And shuddering originates from this sensation. This occurs when the [putrefying] matter is outside the veins.

This fever is also characterised by constant vomiting of bilious matter and by diarrhoea with the colour of gall, especially in the third and fourth bout, and the urine of those who suffer from it will be red, fiery and fine. Another characteristic of this fever is intense blazing heat and a pricking sensation in the liver since the blood is mixed with bile. When this fever is pure, it mostly lasts for twelve hours and its abatement lasts thirty-six hours. Its maximum number of bouts, when it is pure, is seven, which is equal to fourteen days. But if its cycle lasts for more than twelve hours and its bouts are more than seven, it is not pure. If it is not pure but combined with another fever, it exceeds this limit and will last longer; sometimes even it will start in the autumn and only abate in the [next] spring.

This fever is the most dangerous and frightening of all the putrefying ones and most to be feared. The physician should therefore take care not to use warm things lest the yellow bile arises with its sharpness to the brain, so that a tumour occurs in it and the patient gets phrenitis. This is [even] more dangerous than the danger of the fever [itself], and more to be feared. For the yellow bile, because of its lightness, sharpness (and lightness), does not allow for a mistake of the patient or foolishness of the physician. But he should pay attention in the beginning of the disease, and if the strength of the patient is great and helpful [in combating the disease] and the humours move quietly, the nature should be relieved by means of a decoction prepared from plums, tamarind, violet blossoms, and yellow myrobalan, into which the core of purified Indian laburnum and manna have been macerated. The patient should take this according to his strength and age. He should also be relieved by means of juice and pulp of the two kinds of pomegranates pounded with Sulaymān sugar. One may also give him those infusions or drinks which we have stated in our book purge the yellow bile, suppress its sharpness, and brings an end to its boiling. The physician should especially beware of applying these means on the day of the bout [of the disease], lest he brings upon the nature [of the patient] that which withholds it from combating the disease.

On the days of the bouts the patient should be given half a *ratl* of juice of the two kinds of pomegranates, with one ounce of the drink made of violets or plums or juice of a gourd broiled with crystalline sugar. When the heat is strong and the thirst intense, he should only take two *mithqāl*s of fleawort seed with juice of the two kinds of pomegranates and a drink of rose-water syrup. He should be extremely careful not to take food in the time of the bout or in the three hours before it.

If the bout of the fever starts in the morning the patient should only take a drink of rose-water syrup, pomegranate, or plum syrup until the bout of the fever ends. Hereafter he should take broth of fortified barley, and at the end of the day bread pulp boiled several times with water and some pounded crystalline sugar.

If the nature [of the patient] is constipated, and he is unable because of, for instance, corrupt air or lack of strength and the like, to take a preventive medicine in the beginning of the disease, he should be given in the days of the abatement [of the fever] manna from Khurāsān and preserved violets, ten *dirhams* of each; five *dirhams* of the core of purified Indian laburnum without its seed and peel; this should be well macerated in warm sweet water or in juice of broiled gourd and strained; then an ounce of pure plum juice should be added to it. It should be taken in the morning.

On the day of the bout the patient should take mucilage of fleawort seed with juice of the two kinds of pomegranates, a drink made of violets, plums or Sulaymān sugar. If the nature reacts to this and resumes its equibalance by means of this regimen, [it is fine]. But if not, one should administer to him a suppository prepared from violet blossoms, scammony, natron, brown sugar and lycium or a clyster prepared from plums, grapes, sebesten, violet blossoms, husked barley, bran juice, beet juice, oil of violets, sugar, and borax. It should be done carefully and applied in a gentle way.

On the sixth day the patient should adhere to the same regimen as on the days of the bouts [of the fever], so that on the seventh day his body will be completely empty and clean. For then his nature can devote itself to the single task of combating the disease and softening the [putrefying] matter, since it will not be diverted any more by the taking of food or medicine.

If the patient complains during the paroxysm [of the disease] about thirst and a dry uvula and throat, he should drink mucilage of fleawort seed extracted by means of cucumber juice with some oil of violets or by means of juice of a water-melon or of the two kinds of pomegranates. He should chew mucilage of fleawort seed, mucilage of quince seed and oil of violets. Moreover, the water [which the patient drinks] should be mixed for him with a drink made of plums, rose-water syrup, violets or fleawort seed according to the regimen we have mentioned and prescribed in the chapter on cough.[13]

If the inflammation departs from the patient and the acuteness of the fever abates and he complains about a pricking sensation in his stomach, he should be administered bread pulp washed with crystalline sugar. For vegetables he should eat orache, wild-amaranth, cucumber, gourd, or lettuce which should be boiled for him with mungo bean, fresh coriander and almond oil. But he should only take this when the fever has abated and the distress has gone.

When he gets a headache, oil of roses or oil of violets mixed with vinegar should be put on his forehead and temples, his nose should be moistened with oil of nenuphar, oil of violets or oil of gourd seed. When dryness prevails over his brain so that he gets phrenitis, he should have a clyster of one of these oils with the milk of a woman who is breastfeeding a girl. Milk should also be poured over his head, in addition to water in which poppy, lettuce or lettuce seed, violet blossoms and leaves of fleawort have been cooked. His feet should be put in warm sweet water and rubbed with oil of violets. Cold aromatic plants should be put in front of him.

When he suffers from spontaneous vomiting or diarrrhoea on the seventh day because of the activity of his nature, he should

---

[13] Bk. 3, ch. 6.

let it continue as long as he has the strength for it. One should administer to him an ingredient that abates the heat of the stomach and quenches his thirst, such as a drink of unripe, sour grapes, the two kinds of pomegranates, [different] kinds of apples, roses, preserved roses, or plums. [He should drink] water in which *tabashīr*, sandalwood and purslane seed have been steeped for him.

When the diarrhoea becomes so bad that we fear that the patient will lose his strength, we should hasten to treat and stop it by means of inspissated juice of myrtle, quince and *tabashīr* pastilles prepared with sorrel seed and similar cold astringent drugs which we have mentioned in the chapter on diarrhoea.[14] Even so, if he gets *saḥj*[15], faints or suffers from jaundice, it should be treated as we stated in our discussion of that particular affliction in accordance with the opinion of the physician in each particular disease.

Chapter four: On the fever which originates from the blood and which is called "synochous" in Greek

Since blood is by nature the best balanced element, the sweetest in taste, and closest to the temperament of man, nature composed it and made it the substance with which the body feeds itself and by which it subsists. Nature also made it circulate with itself

---

[14] Cf. Bk. 4, ch. 20.

[15] *saḥj*: cf. Lane, Dictionary, p. 1315: "Dysentery, or the like; a certain disease of the bowels; an abrading disease in the belly."

through the whole body, so that the organs can derive their growth from it. For from blood they receive their nutrition and strength and by it they subsist. If blood increases in quantity and its quality is modified, nature will hate it and will cease to regulate it, as a man will hate his child when he stops obeying him, although he is more loved and favoured by him than anyone else. Consequently the blood will remain unripe and undigested; it will pass beyond the limit of balance, change and putrefy. From its putrefaction the fever which in Greek is called "synochous", i.e. continuous, unbroken fever, originates, for the blood is by nature inside the veins and arteries, which are its ways and passages to the whole body.

In his book "On the types of fevers" Galen has adduced clear proof that there are two different kinds of putrefying fevers. One of these is the fever originating from the putrefaction of the humours inside the veins and arteries, and another is the fever originating from the putrefaction of the humours outside the veins [and arteries]. He has also shown that fever is continuous when the putrefaction is inside the veins, and that it is intermittent when the putrefaction is outside the veins. A hot fever may also originate from pure blood that has become warm and inflamed inside the veins and arteries, while the blood is not affected by putrefaction or corruption. This fever is characterised by the fact that it is mostly followed by asthma, since it originates, as we explained, from pure blood that is most strengthful in the heart and lungs. The ancient physicians have therefore surnamed this fever "asthmatic heat", since asthma is mostly caused by the heat of the chest, heart and lungs.

The difference between fever originating from putrefaction of the blood and fever originating from boiling of the blood is that the fever originating from putrefaction is accompanied by a stinking urine and a varying pulsation of the veins, for the contraction of the veins is faster than their expansion. For nature hastens to expel the fumy vapours originating from the putrefaction in a quick way. But fever originating from the boiling of blood is free from these accidents.

Some of the symptoms preceding blood fever and announcing its occurrence are indolence, heaviness and fullness of the members [of the body], a red colour and heat of the surface of the body. Some symptoms following its occurrence are headache, inflammation, a heavy head, swollen temples, bulging eyes, little thirst, much slumber, red phantasms appearing before one's eyes, a fast powerful pulse, red urine verging on purple. This fever is often accompanied by erysipelas and smallpox.

Since this fever originates, as we explained, from a putrefaction of the blood within the veins and arteries, before this disease gets worse and reaches its paroxysm we should see if the strength [of the patient] is healthy, and if his age, temperament, and habit, in addition to the time [of the year] and the nature of the actual weather, are conducive [to restore his health]. When these indications prove to be favourable, especially that of a healthy strength, we bleed the patient and extract a sufficient amount of his blood.

When this disease starts after the patient has consumed a

large amount of food which has collected in his stomach, the venesection should be postponed until the second day or later, so that the nature [of the patient] will be able to digest and cook the food and to expel its superfluity from the bowels and stomach. If the nature does not do this, we do so ourselves by means of a regimen which softens the stomach.

If of all the indications that we mentioned only a healthy strength helps us, we prescribe extracting blood from the patient by means of cupping, instead of venesection. If all the indications help us, except for his strength since it is weak, we should beware of extracting blood by means of venesection or cupping, for it is precisely his strength when it is healthy and firm which combats the disease. We should always observe and consider his strength carefully; we should examine meticulously its health and firmness for combating the disease before we proceed to extracting blood.

If for some reason the extraction of blood in the beginning of the disease is impossible, one should be extremely wary of doing so when the disease is advancing and when it is in its climax. This holds good even if we find the strength [of the patient] to be healthy and good, for in these two phases one should not rely on a healthy strength, since it is engaged with combating and fighting the disease. However, we should extinguish [the burning heat of] the blood and alleviate its sharpness by means of mucilage of fleawort seed, juice of the two kinds of pomegranates and a drink made of pure plum [juice].

If the nature [of the patient] is constipated, one should take ten *dirhams* of purified tamarind, twenty plums, and three *mithqāls* of violet blossoms; this should be boiled in two *raṭls* of water until one half of a *raṭl* is left, it should be strained but not macerated. In that purified substance one should dissolve manna from Khurāsān and core of purified Indian laburnum, ten *dirhams* of each; this should be strained as well, and then the patient should take it.

If the fever was preceded by a disease in the chest or if it occurs simultaneously with it, one should take for that twenty *ḥabbas*[16] of grapes, and five *dirhams* of each of violet blossoms and purlane seed; this should be boiled just like the drug mentioned before; then six *dirhams* of preserved violets, manna from Khurāsān and core of purified Indian laburnum should be dissolved in it; this should be strained and taken.

The patient should be given foodstuff that is fine, quickly digested and of good substance, such as broth of fortified barley or bread crumbs washed several times in water. If the blood is not sharp, the nature [of the patient] should be softened in the beginning with a drug that is cooling and softening, such as juice of roasted gourd in which manna from Khurāsān and core of Indian laburnum has been dissolved; this should be given to the patient.

If the nature [of the patient] responds to this treatment [it is fine], but if not, soft suppositories or clysters should be prepared for him from grapes, sebesten, violet blossoms, husked barley, sugar, violet oil and the like. If the patient is affected by a

---

[16] One *ḥabba* is 0,0446 grams; see Hinz, *op. cit.*, pp. 12-13.

headache the nose should be moistened with violet oil or nenuphar oil; one should take oil of roses, mix it with vinegar and apply it to the forehead and temples. One may also mix oil of roses with rose-water, juice of Egyptian willow, unripe, sour grapes, or purslane, and apply it to the forehead and temples. The hands and feet should be put in water in which camomile and dry violets have been boiled, and one should put bandages on the legs.

If the headache is not alleviated and the chest is free of catarrhs and cough, milk of women or donkeys should be poured over the head, and it should be washed with water in which husked barley, violet blossoms and camomile have been boiled. One should pour oil of violets and nenuphar into his nose. On the head one should put a plaster prepared from purslane juice, gourd peels, mucilage of fleawort seed, barley meal, rose-water and the like.

If the patient is affected by sorrow or if he suffers from an inflammation, one should give him mucilage of fleawort seed extracted with juice of cucumber or with juice of the two kinds of pomegranates. One should also give him water-melon juice with crystalline sugar or rose-water syrup. If lethargy comes over the patient so that he cannot wake up, one should not apply to his head any of the cataplasms or oils which I have prescribed before. However, one should restrict oneself to massage the feet with juice of camomile, violet blossoms and coarsely ground salt. One should rub the forehead and temples with juice of camomile and violet blossoms, and feed the patient with juice of bitter pomegranate with crumbs of fortified bread which has been washed several times in water.

If palpitation occurs to the patient, we apply a plaster to the stomach prepared from sandalwood, rose leaves, barley meal and some camphor kneaded with rose-water, purslane juice or gourd juice. Let him drink rose-water, a potion of pomegranate or rose-water syrup.

If he gets a nosebleed, one should apply to his forehead the plaster that we have prescribed for palpitation. One should pour into his nose juice of green dates or juice of palmtree flowers with some camphor and rose oil. They should be treated with the same regimen as we have mentioned in our description of nosebleeds.[17]

When in the last phase of this fever we need drugs that alleviate and extinguish what is left of it in the body, we use pastilles that we have tested for alleviating blood fever, dissolving the superfluity with fineness, and extinguishing the blazing heat. Its prescription is: Take white *ṭabāshīr*, rubbed yellow sandalwood, purslane seed and inspissated juice of licorice, two *mithqāls* of each; pith of cucumber seed, water-melon seed, and gourd seed, two *dirhams* of each; white gum tragacanth, gum Arabic and starch, one *dirham* of each; cubeb pepper and camphor, two *dāniqs*[18] of each. This should be pounded, sieved and kneaded with mucilage of fleawort seed; then pastilles of one *mithqāl* each should be prepared from it, which should be dried in the

---

[17] Cf. Bk. 2, ch. 15.

[18] The weight of one *dāniq* varies from 0,52 until 0,74 grams.

shade. The patient should be administered one of these pastilles with juice of roasted gourd or with a cold drink. If one wants this drug as an electuary, one should add four *mithqāls* of crystalline sugar, knead it with rose-water syrup and let the patient suck two *mithqāls*, for it is a marvellous and wonderful [remedy], which is also good for erysipelas, measles and smallpox.

Chapter five: On quartan fever

Quartan fever originates from putrefaction of the black bile, for when the putrefied black bile is within the veins and arteries it causes continuous quartan fever, but when it is outside the veins and arteries it causes intermittent quartan fever. It is called quartan fever because it attacks once in every four days for a period of twenty-four hours, and abates for forty-eight hours.

This fever is indicated by the same three things as tertian fever, namely, natural, unnatural and extra-natural. It is indicated by natural things in so far as it mostly happens to someone whose temperament is cold and dry, who is middle-aged, and especially when his body is lean, dry and firm, and his veins thin and concealed. It is indicated by unnatural things in so far as it is indicated by the season of the year when it is autumn, and by the temperament of the actual weather when it is cold and dry, and when the nature of the country is the same. It is indicated by extra-natural things in so far as this fever exposes its patients in the beginning of its bouts and in the beginning of the putrefaction of the [superfluous] matter to a severe cold which exhausts their

bodies and weakens their members. For when the black bile
from which this fevers originates because of its cold and coarseness
streams towards the sensory organs, it makes them heavy and
weak, and crushes them. Someone suffering from it will have a
pale complexion, and his skin will be arid and dry. This fever is
characterised by pain and hardness of the spleen; the urine turns
white, thin and watery in its beginning. At the end of this fever
when the [superfluous matter] becomes soft and fine, the urine
becomes black.

Since this fever originates from the putrefaction of pure black,
cold and dry bile which in turn originates from the burning of
the humours, namely, blood, yellow bile, and phlegm, one should
try to distinguish every single humour according to its
characteristics. For in this way one can moisten it by means of
an appropriate regimen and treatment.

When it is clear from the symptoms mentioned by us that this
fever originates from the putrefaction of pure black bile, we
should treat the patient with ripe things which are quickly
discharged, such as juice of endive, horse-fennel and celery.
One should take half a *ratl* of this altogether, when it has been
boiled and strained, and when one ounce of oxymel syrup prepared
with honey, or when honey prepared with spices has been added
to it. One may also dissolve roses preserved in honey in it and
drink it. Or let him take the decoction of roots or the drink of
absinth.

The [superfluous] matter should be slowly evacuated by means
of vomiting; perspiration should be provoked by means of oil of

camomile, aneth, or water-mint; take care not to empty the body in a rigorous way in the beginning of the disease. When the fever has started to abate and signs of cooking and digestion become visible, we evacuate the black bile with clysters and with drugs which purge that humour, and during this time we administer to the patient pastilles of agrimony, rhabarber, anise and lac, according to the composition which we have mentioned in book five of this work.

In addition to this [treatment] one should give the patient [different] drinks, such as the drink made of lemon-grass, mint, and the decoction of roots. In the end of this disease one should take the theriac known as "fārūq"[19], and the electuary prepared with cumin. One should, however, beware of using these drugs in the summer and in a hot country and at a young age; but they should be used in the winter, in cold countries, at an advanced age and in the case of someone whose temperament is dominated by cold. One should also avoid applying cooling things because they make the matter coarse, prevent it from cooking and thus prolong the duration of the disease.

If this quartan fever has been preceded by tertian fever and the patient is a young skinny man whose temperament is dominated by yellow bile and whose urine is blond, fire coloured, while he suffers from intense thirst and severe insomnia, and it is summer and the nature of the actual weather is hot and dry, we know from these indications that the fever originated from the burning

---

[19] For the composition of this famous theriac see Ibn Sīnā, *op. cit.*, Bk. 5, pp. 310-313; cf. Ullmann, *Medizin*, p. 321.

of yellow bile. In this case it is necessary to treat the patient in the beginning with cooling and softening things, such as juice of the two kinds of pomegranates, oxymel prepared with sugar, and barley broth with juice of the two kinds of pomegranates and oxymel.

If the nature [of the patient] suffers from constipation, we try to soften it with juice of plums, manna, and preserved violets. Or take juice of endive and juice of fennel that has been boiled and strained, macerate core of purified Indian laburnum and manna in it, and let him drink this. If the nature does not respond to this, we prescribe for the patient the application of relieving clysters. If the matter starts to cook and its movement from place to place becomes lighter, one should administer to him a decoction which purges the burned yellow bile without harshness, such as a decoction of plums, tamarind, and manna, and the like.

But one should beware of doing this before the cooking of the matter. The patient should suck [juice of] the two kinds of pomegranates and winter grapes; he should feed himself with mungo beans, wild-amaranth, or orache. When the fever has abated in the end of the disease, he should pour over his body lukewarm water or water in which camomile, melilot and violet blossoms have been cooked. He should rub himself with wine mixed with violet oil.

If this fever is preceded by a disease of the blood, so that the temperament of the patient is, moreover, blood-like and his veins are full and his urine is coarse and red, while he has a sweet taste in his mouth and sleeps much, and it is in the spring season, we know from this that the fever originated from the burning of the blood. In this case it is necessary to apply those means which soften and cook the matter without heating [it], such as oxymel and barley broth prepared with oxymel. One should take preserved roses and preserved violets, macerate them in hot endive juice, strain this and administer it to the patient. One should put his feet in warm water in which camomile and violet blossoms have been cooked. One should make him vomit at the beginning of the bouts and when cold occurs. He should suck juice of the two kinds of pomegranates after it has been mixed with oxymel, and he should eat fine foodstuffs.

When the matter is mature, we hasten to extract blood by bleeding the basilic vein or the median cubital vein, so that the coarse burned blood is evacuated. Hereafter we relieve the nature by means of decoctions which make the blood thin and remove its sharpness and temper its blazing heat. When this fever lasts longer than twenty days we enjoin the patient to fast on every day of its bout and to take light food on the other days.

When this fever is preceded by a phlegmatic disease and the patient is an old man who has a moist and cold temperament, a slow pulse, uncooked, coarse and white urine, and suffers from light sneezing, while the time [of the year] is winter and the nature of the actual weather is cold and moist, we know from from these indications that the fever is caused by burning of the phlegm. In this case one should first of all administer to the patient juice of endive, fennel, and celery, half a *raṭl* altogether. One should boil and purify this and macerate roses and violets preserved in honey in it, ten *dirhams* of each; this should be purified and consumed.

When the nature [of the patient] suffers from constipation, we relieve it by means of juice of bindweed with sugar or by means of a strong clyster which brings the matter down. The patient should rub his body with hot oils which open the pores and attract perspiration. He should abstain from eating on the day of the bout [of the fever] unless his strength is weakened. He should take some food and eat the meat of birds that is soft and tender. He should drink something that is soft and moderately warm.

He should feed himself with juice of chickpeas, oblong pieces of beet and its roots. He should beware of everything that is cooling and moistening. After the meal he should take the cumin-electuary, the electuary prepared with the three peppers, and the anise-electuary. It is good when he vomits either by means of leaves of radish and juice of aneth or by means of oxymel prepared with honey, in which sliced radish has been macerated from the night until the morning. He should take repeatedly the *fārūq*-theriac, the costus, rhabarber and sulphur remedy, and similar electuaries.

When the disease lasts longer than three weeks, he should feed himself with chickens and francolins, and when the fever lasts longer than forty days, he should take the meat of one-year-old lambs. He should take those drugs which open the obstruction, make the urine stream, and strengthen the bowels. This is a brief, concise and yet sufficient account of the treatment of quartan fever caused by putrefaction of the black bile and by the burning of the humours.

Chapter six: On quotidian fever

Quotidian fever originates from the putrefaction of the humoral phlegm. The eminent physicians have explained in their works that every matter, whether it consists of phlegm, yellow or black bile, when it putrefies, acquires [the quality of] cooking (and boiling), and that from this cooking (and boiling) heat and fever originate. Even so the phlegm when it putrefies and is spread throughout the body and is inside the veins and arteries, causes a fever which is called in Greek "amphemerinos", that is "the continuous", for it is not broken and not accompanied by cold.

When the putrefaction of the phlegm is outside the veins and arteries, it causes intermittent fever which abates and attacks every day. The period of its bout is eighteen hours, and of its abatement six hours. This fever is indicated by the same three things as tertian and quartan fever, namely, natural, unnatural, and extra-natural.

It is indicated by natural things in so far as it mostly occurs to someone whose temperament is cold and moist, and whose age is that of an old or young man, because of the domination of the phlegm over old men by nature and over young men by coincidence. It is indicated by unnatural things in so far as it mostly originates in the time of the winter, when the temperament of the actual weather is similar to the nature of the time [of the year] in cold and moisture, and even so the temperament of the country, and especially when the patient while healthy was used to rest, tranquillity, and much comfort, and did not exert or strain himself very much. This fever is indicated by extra-natural things in so far as in the beginning its patients are afflicted by a severe cold similar to a severe frost which makes the whole body cold, even the hands and feet, and lasts for one hour. When the phlegm putrefies and becomes hot, its heat increases slowly, the cold diminishes, and the fever will be light and delicate in its progress. However, it will be protracted and frightening, and accompanied by pain in the stomach. For the phlegm mostly originates in the cardia of the stomach. Its patients will therefore throw up a bilious substance; they will feel nauseous; their faces will be swollen and their complexion will become grey as lead, tending towards whiteness and paleness; their mouths will be moist; in most cases they will not suffer from thirst.

The physician can deduce the quality of treatment of this kind of fever from the nature of the phlegm: one kind of phlegm is the cold and moist one; it is really the natural kind that originates from the pure and watery part of the blood. Another kind of phlegm is that which is more cold and more coarse but less moist like the acid phlegm which originates from the cold dominating the pure and watery part of the blood. Yet another kind of phlegm is that which is more hot and more dry such as the salty phlegm which originates from the heat dominating the pure and watery part of the blood.

When the patient suffers, in addition to the fever, from thirst and a dry mouth, we understand that the fever originates from salty phlegm. In this case we prescribe administering to the patient oxymel prepared with sugar and hot water on an empty stomach. When the bout of the fever arrives and cold occurs, the patient should put his feet in water in which camomile, aneth, and violet blossoms have been boiled; the soles of his feet should be rubbed with salt and violet oil.

When vomiting occurs spontaneously in the beginning of the disease, it indicates that the superfluity is fine and light and that it moves fast. When vomiting does not occur spontaneously and one cannot stimulate it artificially in the beginning of the disease since it is impossible, it indicates that the superfluity is coarse and solid, hard to melt, and slowly moving. The patient should eat roses preserved in sugar, and drink hot water in addition, because hot water is very recommendable in [the case of] this fever, since it will soften, dissolve and melt the [superfluous] matter. One hour after the consumption of the preserved roses, he should take barley broth with oxymel prepared with sugar.

If the nature [of the patient] responds to this [it is fine], but if not, one should give him up to half a *raṭl* of juice of bindweed with one ounce of Sulaymān sugar. One may also dissolve manna from Khurāsān and preserved roses in it, one ounce of each, and strain this and let him consume it. If the nature [of the patient] responds to this [it is fine], but if not, one should prepare a soft clyster or purging suppositories for him.

When the patient remarks that he feels flatulence and rumbling in his bowels or complains about nausea and an upset stomach, we know from this that the [superfluous] matter has melted, is streaming and looking for a way out. As for relaxation [of the bowels] in the case when the patient feels flatulence and rumbling, it is necessary to help the nature to expel the matter softly and gently, by, for instance, administering to the patient a soft reliable decoction or similar pastilles, or purging rose pastilles and the like. If he complains about nausea and an upset stomach we prescribe for him in the beginning of the cold of every bout a drink of oxymel prepared with sugar and juice of aneth when it has been boiled. One should attract vomiting without affecting the stomach in a harsh way.

If the body [of the patient] has not enough strength to bear the purgatives, one should treat him artfully by softening and purifying the [superfluous] matter without affecting the nature [of the patient] harshly. This should be done according to the nature of the matter, according to the element by which it is dominated, and according to the organ towards which the matter is inclining. If the matter consists of salty phlegm and inclines towards the liver, we administer to the patient those drugs that are especially good for purifying the liver, softening the matter and expelling the urine, such as pastilles of *ṭabashīr*, camphor or sandalwood with oxymel prepared with sugar. When the phlegm is acid, he should be administered pastilles of roses or barberry or anise with juice of endive, fennel, and celery, half a *raṭl* altogether, with one ounce of oxymel syrup prepared with honey. [Let him also take] one of the pastilles which we have mentioned [above] and adhere to this kind of regimen for a week.

If the fever is lasting and does not abate with this kind of regimen, one should give the patient the decoction of roots according to the prescription mentioned by us in the fifth book of this work,[20] or a drink of lemon-grass or absinth. If the matter inclines towards the stomach and the phlegm is acid, we should treat [the patient] in the beginning of the disease with a drink of honey and warm water or oxymel syrup prepared with honey and warm water. He should be fed with broiled barley broth with peels of fennel roots and celery roots. When this has been purified, one should add oxymel prepared with honey to it.

When the patient is affected by cold in the beginning of the bout of the fever, one should let him drink aneth juice and oxymel syrup prepared with honey with sliced radish. He should stimulate vomiting and put his feet into water in which camomile, melilot, thyme, and southernwood have been boiled. When vomiting occurs spontaneously, he should not try to stop it especially in the beginning of the disease, and one should administer to him roses preserved in honey with warm water. When the superfluity is mature, one should administer to him an infusion of aloe or an infusion of the electuary with aloe,[21] or an absinth decoction or mastic and aloe pastilles.

When the patient has no strength to bear what we have prescribed, one should give him agrimony, absinth, or rhabarber pastilles with vegetable juice and oxymel syrup prepared with

---

[20] See Bk. 5, ch. 9 (MS Dresden fols. 186-193).

[21] Also called "iyāraj fīkrā," whose main component was aloe, see Ullmann, *op. cit.*, p. 296.

honey. He should stimulate vomiting in the beginning of the bout and refrain from food until the severity of the fever has subsided. He should not strive for a very soft regimen since this fever is protracted and only abates after a long time.

For when he strives for a very soft regimen in the case of a protracted disease, his strength is confounded and weakened. When we see signs of ripeness in the urine, we should apply a warm poultice around the stomach and rub it with ingredients that have a strengthening effect and that remove the superfluities from it, such as oil of nard, mastic, absinth, aneth and the like. One should apply this poultice with water in which violets, nard, mastic and absinth, and the like have been boiled. One should apply packs that are moderately warm and fragrant, and the water should be mixed with exquisite wine or with a drink of honey boiled with spices. One should administer to the patient drugs that are good for someone whose stomach is upset, for this fever is especially characterised by pain in the stomach, as we have explained and elucidated.

GLOSSARY OF MATERIA MEDICA

أترنجّ cedrat → حمّاض

إجّاص plums
114,161,218,219,266,281,292,392,401,407,
418,420,423,436,533,535,664,671 لإجّـــاص

الأسود black plums 283

إذخر lemon-grass 648,811

آس myrtle 179,329 → ربّ

أفاويه → عسل

أفسنتين absinth 638,823,826,836 → دهن

إكليل الملك melilot 676,820

آنيسون anise 646,805

إوز → شحم

إيارج electuary 823

بابونج camomile 110, 121, 135, 559, 562, 571, 573,
676, 686, 771, 820, 836 → دهن

بزر الحمّاض sorrel seed 460

بزر خسّ lettuce seed 310-311

بزر خشخاش poppy seed 311

بزر رجلة   purslane seed 268,457,541,588

بزرقطونا   seed of fleawort 154,266,267,403,437 →

لعاب، ورق

بطّيخ   water-melon → لبّ

البقلة اليمانية   wild-amaranth 176,440,674

بقول   vegetables 440,827

البلح الأخضر   green dates 582

بلّوط   acorn 289

بنفسج   violets 106, 113, 149, 161, 179, 219,265,270,

272,279,284,291,401,414,420,436,532,559 →

نوّار، ورق

بنفسج مربّى   preserved violets 219,279,414,543,665,684

بورق   borax 425

ترنجبين   manna 665,667,671

ترنجبين خـرسـاني،   manna from Khurāsān 219,279,284,414,
537-538,543,549,782-783

التـرياق المعـروف بالفـاروق   the theriac known as "fārūq" 650

ترياق الفاروق   the *fārūq* theriac 716

تفّاح   apple 455

التمر الهندي   tamarind 217-218,283-284,392,534,671

جرادة القرع   gourd peels 301,308,323,564

جلاب   rosewater-syrup 113, 148, 161, 266, 319,326,
404,407,436,568,579,596

the anise-electuary 713 جوارش الآنيسون

the electuary prepared with والجـوارش المتّخـذ بالثلاثة فـلافل
the three peppers 712

the cumin-electuary 712 الجوارش الكمّوني

the electuary prepared with cumin الجوارش المعـمول بالكمّون
650

broth of barley 176,227,261,408,546,663, 683,780,814	حسو الشعير
unripe, sour grapes 118,320,327,329,454,557	حصرم
lycium 287,288,423	حضض
chickpeas 710	حمّص
sorrel ← بزر	حمّاض
cedrat pulp 320,327	حمّاض الأترنجّ

lettuce 311,441,449 ← بزر، قلوب	خَسّ
poppy 449 ← بزر	خشخاش
vinegar 108,329,444,555	خلّ
wine vinegar 300	خلّ خمر
Egyptian willow 106,330,557	خلاف
cucumber 441	خيار
gillyflower 127 ← دهن	خيري

meal of barley 151,307,321,565,577	دقيق شعير
water-melon 180,265,295,433,568	دلاع

دهن 139

دهن الأفسنتين   oil of absinth 834-835

دهن البابونج   oil of camomile 130,640

دهن بنفسج   oil of violets 107,157,159-160,173,289,292,
302,305,312,314,425,433,435,444,445,450-
451,553,554,563,572,677,771-772

دهن الخيري   oil of gillyflower 131

دهن السوسن   oil of lily 131

دهن الشبثّ   oil of aneth 130,640,835

دهن الفوذنج النهري water-mint 640

دهن حبّ القرع   oil of gourd seed 445-446

دهن لوز 442

دهن المصطكى   oil of mastic 834

دهن الناردين   oil of nard 834

دهن نيلوفر   oil of nenuphar 107,157,173,302,311-312,
445,555,563

دهن ورد   oil of roses 108,157,160,300,316,317,323,
444,555,556,582-583

أدهان   oils 129,447,571,706,835

رازيانج   قشور → fennel 634,666,701,805

راوند   rhabarber 645,716,827

ربّ الآس   inspissated juice of myrtle 459

ربّ السفرجل   inspissated juice of quince 459

ربّ السوس   inspissated juice of licorice 588

purslane 115,150,152,176,301,308,322,557,   رجلة

564,578 ← بزر، قضبان

pomegranate 65,116,268,272,273,294,317,   رمّان

seedless الرمّان الإمليس 319,326,407,579

bitter الرمّـــان المرّ pomegranate 263

pomegranate 574

the two kinds of the pomegranates 112,117,   رمّانان
147,154,160,179,394,400,404,419,434,455,5
32,567, 662,673,688

plants 105   رياحين

orache 153,440,675   سرمق

quince ← ربّ، لعاب   سفرجل

scammony 286,422   سقمونيا

145,425,553,704   سكّر

brown sugar 422   سكّر أحمر

Sulaymān sugar 269,395,420,782   سكّر سليماني

crystalline sugar 113,115,148,180,262, 274-   سكّر طبرزد
275,314,326,328,402,439-440,568,595

oxymel 663,683,684   سكنجبين

oxymel 662-663,769,780,793-794,803 سكنجبين سكّري

oxymel prepared with honey 636,714,806, سكنجبين عسلي
814, 816,818,827

oblong أضلاع السلق وأصوله beet 291,425   سلق
pieces of beet and its roots 710

nard 836	سنبل
licorice → ربّ	سوس
lily → دهن	سوسن
gruel of parched barley 274,325	سويق الشعير
aneth 121,135,714,771,794,818,820 → دهن	شبثّ
(medicinal) drink 113,114,149 passim	شراب
(medicinal) drinks 113,153,594,648	أشربة
exquisite wine 838	شراب رفيع
a potion of honey boiled with spices 838	شراب العسل المطبوخ بالأفاويه
barley 272,298 → حسو، دقيق، سويق، عجين	شعير
husked barley 424,553,562	شعير مقشور
aloe 823,824	صبر
gum Arabic 590	الصمغ العربي
sandalwood 178,307,456,577,803	صندل
yellow sandalwood 587	صندل أصفر
the two kinds of sandalwood 321	الصندلان
the decoction of roots 638,649,810	مطبوخ الأصول
149,456,459,802	طباشير
587	طباشير أبيض

طبرزد ← سكر،

duck-weed 150,308,322	طحلب
palmtree flowers 582	طلع
Armenian earth 268	طين أرمني
electuary 595	معجون
717	معجونات
barley dough 278	عجين شعير
lentils 328	عدس
honey 813	عسل
gallnut 65	عَفْص
bramble 290	علّيق
jujube 218,423,541,552	عنّاب
winter grapes 180,264,674	العنب الشتوي
agrimony 645,826	غافت
bread crumbs 273,298,546, 574	فتات (الخبز)
لباب	فقّوص
mint 649	فوذنج
لبّ ← cucumber 319,432,567	قثّاء
pastille 807	قرصة
pastilles 149	أقرصة

أقراص pastilles
459,585,592,645,646,791,802,804,807, 826

قَرْع gourd 115,153,176,278,326,328,402,417,441,

548,578,594 ← جرادة، دهن، قشور، لب

قُسْط costus 716

قشور أصول الرازيانج peels of fennel roots 815

قشور أصول الكرفس peels of celery roots 815

قشور القرع gourd peels 151

قضبان الرجلة purslane stalks 327

قلوب الخسّ core of lettuce 116

قيصوم southernwood 820

كافور camphor 149,152,178,577,582,591,802

كبابة cubeb pepper 591

كبريت sulphur 716

كثيراء بيضاء white gum tragacanth 590

كرفس celery 635,701,805 ← قشور

كزبرة coriander 441

كمّثرى pears 456

لبّ بزر البطّيخ pith of watermelon seed 589

لبّ بزر القثّاء pith of cucumber seed 589

لبّ حبّ القرع pith of gourd seed 589

لبّ خيار شنبر core of Indian laburnum 218,282,393,415,

538,543,549,666

kernels of cucumber 116 لبّ القثّاء

bread pulp 114,228,261,409,439 لباب الخبز

pulp of the green and raw water-melon 264 لباب الفقّوص

bindweed 704,781 لبلاب

milk of a woman who is breastfeeding لبن امرأة ترضع جارية

a girl 447-448

milk 448 ألبان

milk of a donkey 561 ألبان الأتن

milk of women 561 ألبان النساء

mucilage of the seed of fleawort 151,264- لعاب البزرقطونا

265,294,303,308-309,313,318,322-323,419,

432,434,532,564,566,592

mucilage of quince seed 313-314,434- 435 لعاب حبّ السفرجل

mucilages 315 لعابات

lac 646 لك

mungo bean 441,674 ماش

sebesten 424,552 مخيطا

marjoram 121,127,135 مرزنجوش

mastic 824,836 → دهن مصطكى

salt 771 ملح

coarsely ground salt 572 ملح جريش

water, juice 109,112,117 passim ماء

827	مياه
rose-water 152,303,307,315,322,323,556, 565,577-578	ماء الورد
دهن ←	ناردين ←
bran 291,424	نخالة
starch 590	نشاستج
natron 286,293,422	نطرون
thyme 121,820	نمام
violet blossoms 109,392,422,424,449,535, 541,552,562,571-573,677,686,771	نوّار بنفسج
nenuphar ← دهن	نيلوفر
endive 152,634,665,685,700,805	هندباء
roses 106,114,150,152,179,303,307,315,322, 323,330,455,556,557,565,791,804 ← ،دهـن ماء، ورق	ورد
preserved roses 455-456,684,779,783	ورد مربّى
roses preserved with sugar 777	وردا مربّى سكّريا
roses preserved with honey 637,702,822	ورد مـربّى عـسـلي (بالعـسـل)
leaves of fleawort 106,449-450	ورق البزرقطونا

purslane leaves 286   ورق بنفسج

leaves of radish 714   ورق الفجل

rose leaves 307,577   ورق ورد

jasmine 127   ياسمين

GLOSSARY OF TECHNICAL TERMS

إبط → حمّى

أجل 12

أخذ: اتّخذ متّخذ 290,423,551,683,784 391, 285,306,321,
552,564,576 → حمّى

أذي: آذى → حرارة، سبب

أرق 310 وأرقه كثيرا 659

أرنبة → حمّى، ورم

اطريطاوس (τριταῖος) 336

ألم 9 ألما قويا دائما 78 ألم المعدة 755,840

*امفيمارينوس (ἀμφημερινός) 732

مأمون → مطبوخ

أوّل الأوائل 490

باسليق → فَصْد

بخار 83,105,112,121,136 البخار المنحصر 142
بخار عذب 210

بخرات بخرات غريزية حارّة 68 → حصر، طبيعة

ابتداء 193,212,259,548,662,700,751 ابتداء المرض
216,220,225,411,514,641,773,775,813,821
ابتداء العلّة 390,527 في ابتداء كلّ نوبة من
نوائبها 618 ابتداء عفونة المادّة 618-619

ابتداء هذه الحمّى 624 ابتداء النوائب 687
ابتداء البرد من كلّ نوبة 793 ابتداء نوبة
الحمّى 817 ابتداء النوبة 828

مبادرة ← طبيعة

بدن ← 72,244,246,358,471,479,585,612,730,751
برد، حرارة، سطح، مـسامّ، إصـلاح، عروق،
عمق، فرغ، قوّة

أبدان 32, 51, 54, 56, 66, 67, 76, 81, 124, 141, 156,
675, 705 ,159 وأبدانهم على غـاية الخـلاء
والنقاء 428-429 ← تجفيف، دلك، ذبل، سدّ،
ظاهر، مادّة

برد 751 أبـرد 143,294,711 بـرّد 303,548,662 ←
أشياء

بَرْد 57,59,60,63,119,125,340,620,687,733,754,
770,817 البرد الشديد 33 برد الهواء 129 برد
شديد متعب للبدن مفتّت للعظام 619 وفي من
الغالب على مزاجه البرد 653-654 برد شديد
شبيه بالزمهرير 751 ← ابتداء، غلبة، قام

بارد 611,615,742 ← بلدان، بلغم، أدوية، رياحين،
طبيعة، عفونة، مزاج

بريد بريد الموت 12

برودة 747

برسام 331,387,447

برهان	47
براهين	البراهين الواضحة 480-481
أبزن	123
انبساط ←	عرق
بطيء	بطيء الحركة 776-777 ← نبض
بَطْن	517 ← تدبير
باطن	140 باطن الجسد وظاهره 13
بعد	بعد انحلال 830
بلد	183 البلد الحارّ 652 ← مزاج
بلدة ←	طبيعة
بلدان	البلدان الباردة 653
بلغم	629,730,753,756,803,812 تشـــيّط البلغم واحـتـراقـه 699 البلغم البـارد الرطب وعلى الحقيقة وهو النوع الطبيعي 761-762 البلغم الحـامض 764 البلغم المالح 765,768 بلغـمـا مالحا 799-800 ← طبيعة، عفونة، غلبة
بلغماني	728 ← قاء، أمراض
بول	72,802,832 ويكون البول...أبيض رقيقا مائيا 624 صـار البـول أسـود 625 وبوله أشقر ناريا 658 وبوله أحمر غليظا 679 وبوله نيئا غليظا أبيض 696-697 ← أدوية، حمرة، نتن
أبوال	أبوالهم تكون أصبغ صفرة 97 وتكون أبوالهم حمراء نارية لطيفة 374 ← حمر

أبيض ← بول

بياض 758

ترفة 749

ترك 382,453 ← حمّى

ترك 605 ترك الجماع والحركة 175 ← حمّى

تعب 36,363,749 التعب الجسداني 76,155

تعب: أتعب ← سبب

ثقل أثقل 621

ثقْل 60 ثقْل الرأس 503 ← أعضاء

ثياب ← دثر

جبين 443,557,572,580

جبهة 301,304,306,556

جحظ جحظ أعينهم 86 جحظ العينين 503-504

جدري 407,597

جداء ← لحم، لحوم

جرب: جرّب 585

جرع: تجرّع 432,578

مجسّة ← رقّ، قوّة

جسد ← باطن

جفّ 60,62 جفّف: ويجفّف في الظل 593 ← حمّ، مياه

جافّ 56,77,612,765 ← جلود

جفوف وجفوف أجفانهم 87

جفاف 174,312,431 جفاف الفم 767

تجفيف تجفيف ظاهر الأبدان وتكثيفها 34

أجفان ← جفوف

جلب: استجلب 775 مستجلبة للعرق 706 ويستجلب القيء من غير عنف على المعدة 794-795

جلد 143

جلود 64,66,138,622 جلودهم أجفّ وأقـــحـــل 62 وجلودهم قحلة جافّة 622-623 ← كثف

جامد 776

جمر نار

جمع: اجتمع 194

جماع ← ترك

مجاهدة مجاهدة المرض ومصارعته 530-531 ← صحّة، مصارعة، وقت

جهل جهل الطبيب 389

جار: جاور 367 ← عروق، أفضية

جاز جازت هذا الحدّ 381

جوف 515

تجويف ← تجويف الرئة 196

جوّال 470

جوهر غذاء → 545 محمود الجوهر

حبّ ← نقي

حبوب 791

حبس 459

حجامة 520,522

حدّ جاز → 475 حدّ الاعتدال

حدّة 206,369,388 حدّة الحرارة 98 لحدّة العنصر 193 ← دم، مطبوخات، قمع، كسر

حادّ علل → 547

أحداث 207

حدر: أحدر 704 وأحدرنا بعد ذلك الطبيعة 691 ← حقنة

انحدار ← أشياء

حذر 111,125,139,143,212,246,247,384,397,522, 651,673 أن يحـــذر ذلك غـــاية الحـــذر 222-223,528 ويحذر استعمال ذلك غاية الحذر 397-398 ويحذرون غاية الحذر 404

حارّ 207,357,361,685 ← بلد، حمّى، خلط، أشياء، ضمد، طبيعة، عنصر

حرّ 294,587 حرّ المعدة 454

حرارة 44,51,54,55,66,70,71,75,198,255,402,730

حرارة مفرطة 22 الحرارة الغريزية 25 حرارة
الشمس الصيفية 33 حرارة الشمس
50,103 حرارة السموم 56 حرارة مطبقة
مؤذية مقلقة للطباع مهيّجة لها 191-192
الحرارة المطبقة 197 حرارة المعدة 263
الحرارة الربوية 491 حرارة الصدر والقلب
والرئة 492 حرارة سطح البدن 502 ← حدّة،
زوال، شدّة، صعد، معتدل، غلبة، مادّة

حرد	85,88 الحرد الشديد 37
حرّيف	208
حرافة	193,206,370
حرق:	أحرق، احترق ← بلغم، حمّى، أخلاط، دم، زكام، المرّة الصفراء
حرك: حرّك	217 تحرّك 391
حركة	86,669 ← بطيء، ترك، رَطِب، إفراط، فضل، ينبوع
تحريك	تحريك الطبيعة 220,225
أحزان	38
حسّ	8 ← ينبوع
حسّاس ←	أعضاء
أحشاء ←	أدوية
حصبة	597
حصر	ويحصر البخارات 139-140 ← بخار

استحصاف ← كثف

انحطاط   80,251,642 ← وقت

حفظ   299

حفْظ   234 حفظ القوّة 226

حقَن: احتقن   67

حقنة   290,423 حقنة قوية تحدر المادّة إلى أسفل

705 حقنة لطيفة 784

حُقَن   643 حقن ليّنة 552 الحقن المسهلة 668

محكوك   307,588

حكيم   حكيم الطبّ وفيلسوفه 256

إحكام ← دبر

محكم   المحكم الصنعة 227, 408-409, 546,574

حلّ   287,537,542,549,637,783 انحلّ 43 تحلّل

67,81,359 حلّل 124,141,142,779

تحليل   تحليل الفضل 586

انحلال   185 ← بعد، نضج

حلب   448,561

حلْق   432

حلو ← طعْم

استحمام   33 استحمام بالمياه القابضة المجفّفة 61-62

حمّام   82,102,104,122,125,133,136,174 حمّاما

معتدلا في هوائه ومائه 158 حمّاما عذب الماء

معتدل الهواء 172 ← هواء

حمر:احمرّ   وتحمرّ وجوههم 52 وتحمرّ أبوالهم 92

حمرة   73 حمرة وجوه 85-86 حمرة اللون 501 حمرة البول الشبيهة بحمرة الأرجوان 505-506

أحمر ←   بول، أبوال

حامض   803,812 ← بلغم

حمل: احتمل   221,453,796,825 حمّل على, 304,306,320,324, 443,555,557,580

حملان   لحم

حمي   43,486,753

حمّى   11,29,54 passim حمّى يوم 15,21,22,40, 45, 49,69,74, 76, 79,85, 90 الحمّى التابعة لأورام الأرنبة وأورام الإبط والعنق 41-42 الحمّى المحرقة 189-190,198- 199,204,343,348 هذه الحمّى أعني المحرقة 259 حمّى الغبّ 335,336, 353,608,657,738 حمّى الغبّ ذات النوائب التي تأخذ وتترك 339 حمّى غبّ دائمة 341,343-344,351 حمّى قوسوس أعني المحرقة 341-342 الحمّى المتولّدة من الدم 466 الحمّى التي تسمّى ...سونوخوص أيّ حمّى دائمة وهي المطبقة 477 حمّى العفونة 481 حمّى حارّة 486 الحمّى المتولّدة عن عفونة الدم -493 495 الحمّى المتولّدة عن غليان الدم (وفورانه) 493-494,498 حمّى الدم 500 ولمّا كانت هذه

الحمّى متولّدة عن عفونة الدم 508 حمّى الربع
738، 721، 604، 600، 599 حـمّى الربع الدائمـة
602 حـمّى الربع الدائرة ذات النوائب 603
الحمّى الربعية 657 لحمّى النائبة كلّ يوم 725
هذه الحـمّى التي تنوب كلّ يوم 726 الحـمّى
الدائرة ذات النوائب التي تترك وتأخذ في كلّ
يوم 735-734 ← ابتـداء، تدبيـر، دلائل، دور،
زوال، سبـب، أسـبـاب، سكن، سكون، صلب،
طبيعـة، أعراض، انقضاء، كسر، انكسار،
كيفية، مرار، منتهى، نوبة، نوائب، هزم ، وقت،
أوقات

حمّيات   17,18,243,246 حمّيات العفن 383

حال: استحال   337,472,476

حار   224 حارت القوّة وضعفت 832 تحيّر: تحيّرت
الطبيعة 223-224

حيات   ينبوع

أخبصة   570

خرج: استخرج   264,319,432,433,567 أخرج: وأخرجنا له من
الدم 513

خارج   خارج(ة من) العروق والأوردة (والأوراد) 338،
602-3,734 خـارجة عن (من) العروق 371,485

خارج العروق 483 ← أشياء

إخراج 517,801 إخــــراج الدم 520,522,526,527,689

إخراج المادّة بلطافة ورفق 789-790

خريف 382,615

خياشيم 107,445 ← رطب، زكام

خشونة 313

اختصار ← طريق

خطاء ← خطاء العليل 389

خطر 12,211,383,387

خفّ 669

خفّة 388 ← فضل

تخفيف ← وتخفيف طعامه 693-694

خفقان 318,576,581

خالص 204-206,377,378,380,381 ← دم، عفونة

خلط 293,315,317,323,556 خالط 210

خَلَط 644 الخلط الحارّ الصفراوي 345

أخلاط 390,628 احتــراق الأخلاط وتشــيّطها 628

احتراق الأخلاط 722 ← مصابّة، عفونة

خلا عن 473

خلاء 324 ← أبدان، عمل

خاف   مخوف 755

خوف   211,384,385,387

خيالات   خيالات حمر ترى نصبة العينين 504-505

دبر: دبّر   186,437,633 ويدبّر بإحكام   425 ← عسل

تدبير   333,427,473,583,631,721,797,808,809,829,831

التدبير النافع لأصحاب هذه الحمّى 48 تدبير
المرض 224 تدبير غذاء المريض 231 التدبير
الرطب 243 التدبير اللطيف 261 التدبير المليّن

للبطن   518 ← طبيعة

دثر   ويدثّرون بالثياب 128

داخل   داخل العروق والأوراد (أوردة) 340-341,345-
          346,478,482,486-487,508,601,731   داخـل(ة)
          العروق 199-200,484

درّ: أدرّ ←   أدوية

درّاج   117,177,719

دعا: استدعى   ويستدعى العرق 639 ويستدعى القيء 686
          ويستدعوا القيء 827-828, 819

دقّ   287,394,591

دلّ   773,776 استـدلّ608,49,353,355,359,363,607,
          610,613,614, 616,737,741,744,749

دليل   85

دلائل 58،93،353،365،512،519،521،607،632،660،681،
698،737،832 دلائل حمّى يوم 187

دلالات 101

دلك 316،771 يدلكوا أبدانهم فيه دلكا رفيقا 137

دم 42، 70، 71، 472، 478، 489، 547، 628 إنّ الدم لمّا كان أعدل العناصر طبعا وألذّها طعما وأقربها من مزاج الإنسان 468-469 الدم الخالص 486 الدم النقي 489 تطفئة الدم وتسكين حدّته 531-532 احتراق الدم 681 ليستفرغ غليظ الدم ومحترقه 690 صفو الدم ومائيته 763، 764-766 ← حمّى، خرج، إخراج، إدمان، رونق، سكن، مطبوخات، أمراض، ممازجة

دموي ← مزاج

مدمج 612

دماغ 386

أدمغة 52 ← يبس

إدمان إدمان المشي 36 إدمان الفكرة 38 الإدمان على الأغذية الحارّة والأشربة المسخّنة للدم 39-40

دور دور هذه الحمّى 376

أدوار 378،380

دائر ←   حمّى

دام   صلب ← 203

دائم   حمّى ← 346,484,732

دوى: داوى   185

دواء   الدواء المانع 412   224,288,430,716

أدواء   الأدواء الظاهرة 7,8   4,18

أدوية   الأدوية البـــاردة القـــابضـــة 287,644,651,800
460-461 الأدوية ألتي تفتح السدد وتدرّ البول
وتقوّي الأحشاء 720-721 الأدوية المسهلة 796
الأدوية النافعة لمن به فساد المعدة 839

ذبل   وتذبل أبدانهم 92

ذابل   77

ذهاب   ذهاب الحمّى 148

ذاب   788 أذاب 779

ذوبان   ممتنع الذوبان 776

رئة   490 ← تجويف، حرارة، عروق

رأس   ضمد ← 561,570

روس   50,55,109,111,129,448

ربع ←   حمّى

ربيع   زمان ← 382

ربو	أسباب ← 488
مربّى ←	بنفسج
أرجل	تنزل أرجلهم في ماء 135,819-120,134 وتدخل أرجلهم في ماء حارّ عذب 450 أنزلوا أرجلهم في ماء 770
رجلان	وتنزل رجلي العليل في مـــاء حـــارّ 685 ← أطراف، يدان
رخص	709
رسوم	80
رشّ	330
رصاصي ←	ألوان
رضّ	621
رطب: أرطب	106,171,293,445,630,711 الأشـــيـــاء المرطبــة رطّب: ترطيب الخياشيم 554 مرطوب 182-181 ← شيخ
رَطِب	742,759 رطبة الحركة 754 ← بلغم، طبيعة
رطوبة	56,747,763 رطوبة عذبة 210
رطوبات	124
رعدة	88,340
رعاف	580,583
رعى: راعى	524
رفع: ارتفع	84
رفق	إخراج

رقّ	وترقّ مجستّهم 92 ← مادّة
رقي	385
رونق	رونق الدم وحسنه 58-59
راح: ارتاح ←	نظر
روح	الروح الحيواني 24,43-44 الروح النفساني 25 الروح الطبيعي 26,70
أرواح	13,15,23,24
روائح	روائح ذكية 127
راحة	156
ريحان	330
رياحين	رياحين الخضـرة 169 ويفـرش بـين أيديهم الرياحـين البـاردة 105 ويجـعـل بـين أيديهم رياحين باردة 451
رياضة	الرياضة المعتدلة 140
ريق	على الريق 769
زكام	110 زكام حارّ محرق للخياشيم 53
زمان	697 زمان الصيف 208,360 الزمـان الصيفـي 208 والزمـان مع ذلك صـيـفـا 659 والزمـان فصل الربيع 680 زمـان الشـتـاء 745-746 ← سعد، طبيعة
زمهرير	57,63,119 ← بَرْد
زال	754 أزال ← أشياء، التهاب

زوال	زوال الحرارة 117 زوال الحمّى 442
زاد	209,417,472
سبب	16,18,35,186,655 سبب الحمّى 99 السبب المؤذي للنفس المتعب لها 165
أسباب	12,31,47 أسباب ظاهرة 32 أسباب حمّى يوم 45-46 أسباب الربو 491
سبات	568 ← كثرة
سحج	462
مسحوق	262,270,293,410
سخن	50,66 أسخن 22,43,683 تسخن إسخانا معتدلا 130
ساخن	765
سدّ	يسدّ مسامّ الأبدان 139 ويسدّ مسامّه 144
سدد ←	أدوية
سرعة	86 فضل، نبض
سريع ←	نضج، انهضام
سطح	سطح البدن 81
سعد: ساعد	390,519,521 مساعدة السنّ والمزاج والزمان 510-511
سعط	302,447,563,581
سعال	437,561 السعال اليابس 332
سقط ←	قوّة

112,145,147 passim	سقى
560 سكّن 105,263,454,584 تسكين النفس	سكن
وتلذيذها 166-167 تسكّن غليانها 397 تسكين	
حمّى الدم 586 ← دم	
91	ساكن
249,377,736,748 سكون الحمّى 104	سكون
ومسامّ بدنه 358 ← سدّ، فتح	مسامّ
33,103 ← حرارة، وهج	سموم
السمك النهري 163	سمك
358 ← طبيعة، وقت	سنة
182,357,611,742 وسنّ الشـــبــاب 652 سنّ	سنّ
الشيخوخة 653 ← سعد، غلبة، مقدار	
97,310	سهر
391,394,396,644,670,791 ← حُقَن	سهل: أسهل
205,209	سَهْل
788 إسهال 452,461 الإسهال المصبوغ بالمرّة	إسهال
373 فإن أفرط الإسهال 458 ← أدوية، فتل	
315	سواد
728	سوداوي
104 سورة المرض 277 ← صعود، انقضاء،	سورة
وقت	
وتشدّ الساقان بعصائب 305-306,559 ←	ساقان
قدمان	

سونوخوس (σύνοχος) 467 ← حمّى	
سال	788
شابّ	شابًا نحيفا 658
شباب ←	سنّ
شبّان	207
شتاء	652,697 ← زمان
شحم	395
شدّ	اشتدّ 202 ← ساقان
شدّة	260 شدّة الحرارة 375
شديد	191,403 ← بَرْد، حرد، عطش
شرب	178,418,539,544,550,638,667,685,703,778,
	783,793
أشربة	396 ← إدمان، أغذية
شريانات	اتّصال
شغل	399,430 ← تشاغل 167
شَغْل	530
أشقر ←	بول
شاكل	746
شمّ	126,178,311
شمس ←	حرارة، وهج
شنأ ←	طبيعة
شاب	مشوب 205,209

شوى 278,402,417,548,594

شاط: تشيّط ← بلغم، حرق

أشياء الأشياء الطبيعية، 739-738,610,608,356,354

741 الأشياء التي ليست بطبيعية- 354,359

الأشـــــياء 745-744,739,614-613,609,360

الخــارجــة من (عن) الطبـيــعــة- 355,363

364,610,617,739-740,749-750 الأشياء الحارّة

385 الأشياء المنضجة السريعة الانحدار

634-633 لأشياء المبرّدة 654 أشياء مـقـوّية

مزيلة للفضول 834-833

شيخ 743 شيخا مرطوبا 696

شيخوخة ← سنّ

مشائخ ← غلبة

شياف 285,422

شيافات 552

صبّ 108,137,448,675 انصبّ 621

مصابّة ومصابّة الأخلاط 74

صبي 743

صبيان ← غلبة

صحّة 362,525,748 صحّة القوّة، 520-519,512,510

530 صحّة القوّة وثباتها هي المجاهدة للمرض

523-522

صحيح 529

صَدْر 540,560 → حرارة

صداع 52,110,300,443,503,554,560

صدغان → ورم

أصداغ 108,302,304,306,444,556,558,573,581

مصارعة مصارعة المرض ومجاهدته 192 مصارعة

المرض 399 → مجاهدة، طبيعة

تصرّف تصرّف العليل 362

صعب 204,205

صعوبة 260

صعد: تصاعد تصاعدت حرارته 753

صعود صـعـود المرض 223 صعـود المرض وبلوغـه

سورته 509-510 صعود المرض ومنتهاه 528

صفر: اصفرّ وربّما اصفرّت ألوانهم 87-88

صفرة → أبوال

أصفر → مرّة

صفراء 368

صفراوي 728

صفا: صفّى 280,417,537,539,544,636,666,685,701,703,

783,816

صفو 280,537 → دم

صلب صلبت الحمّى ودامت 200

صلابة → طحال

إصلاح	إصلاح النفس 170 إصلاح البدن 171
صنعة ←	محكم
صورة ←	كيفية
صوم	ألزمنا العليل الصوم في كلّ يوم نوبة 693
صيف	زمان ← 651
ضرّ	13
ضرب	29,108,444,677 ضرّب 300,555
ضعف	حار ← 297,707,825
ضُعْف	ضعف القوّة 221,413
ضعيف	521
ضمد: ضمّد	150 ويضمّد الرأس بضماد 563 ضمّدنا المعدة بضماد 576 وتضمّد بضمادات حارّة معتدلة عطرية 837
ضماد	306,310,321,581 ضمّد ←
ضيّق ←	عروق
طبّ ←	حكيم
طبيب	99,220,230,389,464 ← جهل
أطبّاء	أفاضل الأطبّاء 727
متطبّب	212,384,760
طبخ	109,120,135,328,441,448,536,542,562,676, 686,770,794,815,819,836,838

مطبوخ   790 مطبوخا لطيفا مأمونا 391,670,671,823

مطبوخات   المطبوخـات التي ترقّق الدم وتزيل حـدّتـه

وتكسر وهجه 691-692

طَبْع   207,209 ← دم، غلبة

طباع   على مجرى الطباع 478 حرارة، فعل

طبيعة   216,226,365,391,398,469,473,516,518,547,

789,798 فإن كان في الطبيعة (تعذّر و)امتنا ع

277,534,664 فإن أجابت الطبيعة 285,290,551,

784 طبيـعة الهواء الحـاضر 361,511 طبيـعة

العنصـر المولّد للحـمّى 365-364 وإن كـانت

الطبيعة متعذّرة 411 فإن أجابت الطبيعة

واعتدلت بهذا التدبير 421-420 وتنفرد الطبيعة

بمصـارعـة المرض وتلطيف المـادّة 430-429

شنأته الطبيعة...كما يشنأ المرء ولده إذا خرج

عن طاعتـه 474-473 مبـادرة الطبيـعـة إلى

إخراج البخارات الدخانية 497 طبيعة الفصل

من السنة 614 طبيعة البلدة 616 وطبيعة الهواء

الحـاضـر حارّة يابسـة 660-659 فإن لم تجب

الطبيـعة بذلك 667 وطبيـعة الهواء الحاضر

باردة رطبة 698-697 فإن تعذّرت الطبيعة 704

طبيعة الزمان 747-746 طبيعة البلغم 761 فإن

كانت الطبيعة مجيبة 781 طبيعة المادّة والغالب

عليها 798 طبيعة العضو الذي المادّة مائلة

إليه 799 ← حــدر، حــارّ، تحــريك، أشـيـاء،
نشاط، وقت

مطبق   199 ← حرارة، حمّى

طحال   وجع الطحال وصلابته 623

طرب: أطرب ← ملهى

أطراف   أطراف اليدين والرجلين 752

طريق: طريق مداواتها 9 طريق الاختصار 187

طعم   573

طَعْم   وطعم فمه حلوا 680 ← دم

طعام   706,708,711 طعام كثير 514 ← هَضْم

طفأ: أطفأ   584

تطفئة ←   دم

طلي   129

طوع   452,773,774,821 طوعا

طاعة ←   طبيعة

طال   وطال لبثها 381 متطاول 755

طول   طول مدّة المرض 656,831 طول مدّة 830

طير   709

طيش   388

ظاهر   ظاهر أبدانهم 55,59 ← باطن، تجفيف، أسباب

عجن   288,311,592,596 معجون بـ 152,307,322,577

عدل: اعتدل ← طبيعة

معتدل معتدل المزاج 178 معتدل الحرارة 709 ← حمّام، ضمد

اعتدال ← حدّ

أعدل ← دم

عذر: تعذّر ← طبيعة

عرض عرض تابع لمرض 40-41 ← غلبة

عارض(ة) 463,540

عوارض 96

أعراض 231,364,365,499 الأعراض اللازمة لهذه الحمّى 197

عرق 78,79,82,83 أعرق 124

عَرَق ← جلب، دعا

عِرْق انقباض العرق إلى داخل اسرع من انبساطه إلى خارج 496-497

عروق عروق فم المعدة 195,202 العروق المجاورة للقلب 201,348-349 عروق فم المعدة والكبد والرئة 349 عروق سائر البدن 350 عروق البدن 352 وعروقه ضيّقة خفية 612-613 وعروقه ممتلئة 679 ← خارجة، داخل، عفونة، أفضية، نبض

عصائب ← ساقان

عضو ← طبيعة

أعضاء	الأعضاء الباطنة 4,9 الأعضاء الحسّاسة 367,369,621 ثقل الأعضاء وامتلائها 501 ← مدّ
عطش	759
عَطَش	153,203,403,431,767 عطش شـديد دائم 191 العطش الدائم 197-198 وعطشـه شـديدا 658-659 وعطشه قليلا 697 ← قطع، قلّة
عظم ←	قوّة
اعظام ←	برد
عفن	476,729,730,753 تعفّن 43,337
عفونة	23,338,340,476,484,485,487,498 عـفـونة الأخـلاط داخل العروق والأوراد 482 عـفـونة الأخـلاط خـارج العـروق 483 عـفـونة المرّة السوداء 600,722 عفونة المرّة السوداء خالصة وهي البـاردة اليـابسـة 627 عـفـونة مـرّة سوداء خـالصة 633 عفـونة كيموس البلغم 726-727 عفونة البلغم 734 ← ابتداء، حمّى
عَفَن	185 حمّيات
عليل	147,217,300,310,312,318,329,386,431,512, 633,644,657,661,668,696,700,748,767,769,777 ,786,790,792 ← خطـاء، رجـلان، تصـرّف، صوم، قوّة، مزاج
علّة	540,649,675,718

علل 257 العلل الحادّة 230

علج: عالج 185,462,583,661,813

علاج 141,333,459,631 ← كيفية

أعلام 100

علامات 366,502 علامات النضج والانهضام 642-643

عُمْق عمق البدن 84

عمل 592 معمول 326,460 استعمل 144,181,214-
215,238,289,293,385,423,425,531,551,554,585
648,651,652,654,668,682,708,720, ويستعمل
خلاء المعدة...من الغذاء 295-296 ونستعمل
استقصاء النظر 524-525 ← حذر

عنصر عنصر حاد ناري صفراوي 194 العنصر
الحارّ الصفراوي 366-367 ← حدّة، طبيعة

عناصر ← دم

عنق ← حمّى

عادة 183,252,511

عاق 220,221,412

عينان 94 ← جحظ، خيالات، غور

أعين 90 ← جحظ، فَتْح

غبرة ← لون

غثي 757

غثيان غثيانا وتقلّبا في معدته 787,792

غذا   غـــذّى 240,326,328,440,674,710,718,814 ,114

تغـــذّى 115,177,230,239,251,471 116,161,175

أغذى 244 اغتذي 252

غذاء   70,152,235,244,247,248,271,324,405,430,

545,688,828 الغـذاء السـريع الانهـضـام

المحـمـود الجـوهـر 226–227 ← تدبيـر، عمل،

قدر، كيفية، مادّة

أغذية   إدمـان الأغـذية والأشـربة الحـارّة 69 لأغذية

السـريعة الانهـضـام 144-145 الأغذية الحـارّة

146 الأغذية المرطبة لأبدانهم 161

غسل   561 مـغــســول ,115,261,267,273,274,298,325

409,439,546,574 اغتسال 132

غسلة، غسلات   274,325,547

غشي   332,462

غضب   85,89,166

غلب ←   طبيعة، يبس

غلبة   غلبـة البلغم على سنّ المشـائح بالطبع وعلى

سنّ الصبيان بالعرض 743-744 غلبـة البرد

764 غلبة الحرارة 766

غلْظ   620 ← فجاجة

غَليظ   776 ← بول، دم

غلى   635 غلّى 666,701

غليان   729 ← حمّى، سكن

غمّ: اغتمّ	93
غمّ	90,95,96,166,566
غمز	305,450
غَمْز	174 غمز القدمين 571
غور	غور العينين 95
غائر	91
غار: تغيّر	472
غيظ	166
فتح	ويفتح مسامّها 124,138,141-142 فتّح: مفتّحة للمسامّ 706 ← أدوية
فَتْح	فتح أعينهم 569
فتر	198,203,293
فترات	485 ← أوقات
فتل	288 فتل مسهلة 785
فجّ: فجّج	655
فجّ	فجًّا غير منهضم 475
فجاجة	فجاجة الفضل وغلظه 222
فراريج	117,162,177,718
فرح: فرّح ←	ملهى
فرد: انفرد ←	طبيعة
أفرط ←	إسهال
إفراط	إفراط الحركة الجسدانية 36 إفراط الحركة

النفسانية 37,164

فرغ: استفرغ   217,222,643 وتستفرغ المادّة 639 ولا يستفرغ
البدن...استفراغا عنيفا 641 ← دم

فزع   89

فسد ←   هواء

فساد   487 ← أدوية

فصد   512

فَصْد   515,521,522 بالفـصـد من الـبـاسليق أو من
الأكحل 689-690

فَصْل ←   زمان، طبيعة

مفاصل   78

فَضْل   120,517,776,822 لطافة الفضل وخفّته وسرعة
حركته، 773-774 ← تحليل، فجاجة

فضول   217,246 ← أشياء

أفضية   أفضية العروق المجاورة للقلب 194-195

فعْل   فعل الطباع 453

أَفعال: الأفعال الطبيعية 14

فكرة ←   إدمان

فم   312,316 فم المعـدة 349,756 ← جفـاف، طَعْم،
عروق

أفواه   759

فات   220,225,411

فوران   375,729 ← حمّى

فيلسوف ← حكيم

قانون القانون الصناعي 10

قبح وتقبح ألوانهم 92-91

قبض 144

قابض ← استحمام، أدوية، مياه

انقباض ← عرق

قبل: قابل 165,166

قحل 60,77 ← جلود

قدر: قدّر يقدّر ذلك فيهم على قدر 182 يقدّر الغذاء 237

مقدار 299 مقدار القوّة من المرض 232,233 مقدار مدّة المرض 232,236-237 مقدار القوّة والسن 394 مقدار نوبتها 604-605 مقدار مدّة نوبتها 736

قدمان 771 وتدخل القدمان والساقان في ماء حارّ عذب 304-305 ← غمز

قراقر 786,789

قشر:مقشور ← شعير

قشْر 65,328 ← نقي

قَشعريرة 340,371 قشعريرة صعبة 368

قصب ← نقي

قصر اقتصر على 111,403,406,571

استقصاء ← عمل

قضى: انقضى   104,260,625 انقـضـاء سـورة الحـمّى 134
تنقضي نوبة الحمّى 407-408 انقضاء النوبة
408 تنقضي سورة الحمّى 829

قطع   ويقطع العطش 454

تقعّر   تقعّر الكبد 195,202

قلّ   وتقلّ نضارة وجوههم 91

قلّة   قلّة العطش 504

قليل ←   عطش

قلب   44,71,490 → حرارة، عروق، أفضية، اتّصال،
أوعية، تقلّب ← غثيان

قلق: أقلق ←   حرارة

قمع   وقمعه لحدّتها 255 وتقمع حدّتها 397

قوسوس (καῦσος) 190 ← حمّى

قام: قاوم   إذا كانت هي المقاومة للمرض 234 لمقاومة برد
السحر 255 مقاومة المرض 525

قوام   470,471

قوي: قوّى   209,281,298,472 ← أدوية، أشياء

قوي   402,516

قوّة   34,235,297,299,453,490,521,524,529,707
القوّة الجاذبة والماسكة والهاضمة والدافعة
27-28 وقوّة مجسّتهم وعظمها 87 قوّة العليل
182,390,825 وخفنا على القوّة أن تسقط 458
قوّة البدن 796 ← حفظ،حار، صحّة، ضعف،

مقدار، نبض

قوّى   القوّى النفسانية 14 ← ينبوع

قاء: تقيّاً   713 يتقيّؤون قيئًا بلغمانيا 757

قيء   452,639,773,774,820   الـقــيء المرّي 372 ←

جلب، دعا، امتناع

كبّ: انكبّ   121 انكباب 112,136

كبد   71,150,324,800,801 ← عروق، تقعّر، نخس

أكباد   75

كثرة   كثرة السبات 504

كثف: تكاثف   لتكاثف جلودهم واستحصافها 67-68

تكثيف ←   تجفيف

أكحل ←   فَصْد

كدّ   362

كرب   442

كره   كرها 775

كسر: انكسر   732 انكسرت حدّة الحمّى 438 ← مطبوخات

انكسار   انكسار الحمّى 676-255,675-109,254 ← وقت

كسل   501

كفاية   على قدر الكفاية 513

كمّية   472

كمّد   833,836

كمودة   622,759 ← لون

كهل ‏611

كيفية ‏473 كيفية المرض 233,241-242 كيفية غذاء
المرضى 256 كيفية علاج هذه الحمّى
وصورتها 760-761

كيموس ‏كيموس صفراوي 337 ← عفونة

لبث ← ‏طال

لحم ‏709 لحم الجداء 177 لحم الحملان الحولية
719-720

لحوم ‏لحوم الجداء 162

لَدْغ ‏370 واشتكى لدغا في معدته 439

لذّ: لذّذ ← ‏سكن

لذيذ ← ‏دم

لزم ← ‏أعراض

لسان ‏313,315,316

لطف: لطّف ‏662,682,688,779 ← مادّة

لطافة ‏239,426,586 لطافة النسيم 254 ← إخراج،
فضل

لطيف ‏545,709 ألطف 829,831 ← أبوال، حــقنة،
مطبوخ

تلطيف ‏548,801 ← طبيعة

لمس: التمس ‏156

لهب: التهب ‏56,486 ألهب 70

التهاب   348,351,503,566 فإذا زال عن العليل الالتهاب
438

لهوات   431

ملاه   الملاهي المطربة المفرّحة 168

لون   لون الغبرة والكمودة 59 ← حمرة

ألوان   58,622 وتصــير ألوانهم رصــاصـيـة 758 ←
صفر، قبح

لان: ليّن   138,277,547,664 ← تدبير

ليّن   709

مدّ: استمدّ   لتستمدّ منه الأعضاء 471

مادّة   23,350,371,655,668,682,689,728,787,799,
801,812 مادّة الحرارة الغريزية 25 مادّة لغذاء
الأبـدان 469-470 ولـطـفـت المادّة ورقّت 625
تلطيف المادّة وتنقيتها 797 ← ابتداء، حقنة،
إخراج، طبيعة، فرغ، نَضْج

مداوات   5 ← طريق

مدّة ←   طول، مقدار

مرّة ←   إسهال، ممازجة

المرّة الصفراء   373,385-386,388,396-397,629 احتــراق مــرّة
صفراء 661 المرّة الصفراء المحترقة 670

المرّة السوداء   620,627,643 عفونة المرّة السوداء المتعفّنة 601

مرار   199,200,201 مرار أصفر 206,210 المرار المولّد

للحمّى 347

مرخ   156,159,705,833 تمريخا رفيقا 156 تمرّخ
172,677

مرس   279,393,417,666,684,702 يمرس ذلك...مـرسا
جيّدا 416

مَرْس   537

مرض   30,31,530 → ابتداء، مجاهدة، تدبير، سورة،
صحّة، مصارعة، صعود، طبيعة، طول،
عرض، مقدار، قام، كيفية، نهى، منتهى، وقت

أمراض   12 بعض أمراض الدم 678 بعض الأمـراض
البلغمانية 695

مريض   235,251,252,365,514 → تدبير

مرضى   230,464 → كيفية

مزج   145,303,435,688,837 امتزج 381

ممازجة   لمازجة المرّة الدم 375-376

مزاج   207,357,611,742 ومـزاجـه الطبيـعي 182-183
مزاج البلد(ة) 361,747 مزاج الهواء الحاضر
615,746 ومـزاجـه صـفـراويا 658 وكـان مـزاج
العليل...دمويا 678-679 ومـزاجـه بـاردا 696 →
برد، دم، سعد، عدل

مسح   107,289,301,572

مشي →   إدمان

مص   116,179,263,673,687

مضمض: تمضمض 313,434

معدة   ← ألم، جلب، حـرّ، حـرارة، 293,324,812,833

أدوية، ضمد، عمل، غثيان، فم، لدغ

مَعَد   322

أَمَعاء   517,786

امتلاء   أعضاء ← 111

ممتلئ ←   عروق

مالح ←   بلغم

منع   ← 221,821,828 امـتـنـع 221,569,654,655,706

دواء، طبيعة

امتناع   امتناع القيء 775

ماء   الماء الفاتر 159 الماء العذب الحارّ 330,409,562

173 ← حمّام، أرجل، رجلان، قدمان، يدان

مياه   35 المياه النطرونية والشبّية والكبريتية 34

المياه القابضة المجفّفة 133-132 ← حمّ

مائية   مائية الدم 74 ← دم

نبض   نبض العروق 495 قوّة النبض وسرعته 505

ونبضه بطيئا 696

نَتْن   نتن في البول 495

نحيف   شابّ ← 358,612

نَخْس   370 نخس كنخس الإبر والشـوك 368 نخس

في الكبد 375

نخل 592

نداوة 81,83

نزل: أنزل ← أرجل، رجلان، مطبوخات، يدان،

نزلة 125 ← نضج

نوازل 560,719

نسيم ← لطافة

نشاط نشاط الطبيعة 254

نشف: نشّف 56

نصب 36,363,749

نضج 689,822 أنضج 119,682 ← أشياء

نَضْج 655,669,832 نضج النزلة وانحلالها 126 نضج المادّة 673 ← علامات

إنضاج ← هَضْم

نضارة ← قلّ

نظر 389,510

نظر 237 والنظر إلى الأشـــيــاء التي ترتاح لهـا النفس 168-169 ← عمل

تنظيف 801

نفخ 786,789

نفس ← سبب، سكن، إصلاح، نظر، هموم

نافع ← أدوية

نفا 166

نقصان 243

نقع	64,456 أنقع 714
نقوعات	395
نقيع	65,283,823
انتقال	669
نقّى :نقي	534,538,543,666 منقّى من قــصــبــه وحــبّــه
	282-283 منقّى من حبّه قشره 415 ← مادّة
نقي ←	دم
نقاء ←	أبدان
منهج:	المنهج الطبّي 9
نهى: انتهى	إلى أن ينتهي المرض على التدريج 241
منتهى	238-240 منتهى الحمّى 75 منتهى حمّاهم 79
	منتهى المرض 238 ← صعود
نوبة	373,379,405 نوبة الحمّى 406 ← ابتداء، صوم،
	قضى، مقدار، وقت، أوقات، يوم
نوائب	400 نوائب الحــمّى 249 ← ابتـداء، حــمّى،
	أوقات، أيام
نار ←	نار جمر 128
ناري ←	بول، أبوال
نال: تناول	409,707,711,779
نوم	ونومه كثيرا 680
نيء ←	بول
هبج: تهبّج	وتتهبّج وجوههم 757-758

هدوء   156

هزم   وانهزمت الحمّى 120 انهزام 134

هَضْم   هضم الطعام وإنضاجه 516-517

انهضم ←   فجّ

انهضام   سريع الانهضام 545 ← علامات، غذاء، أغذية

همّ: اهتمّ   93

همّ   90,95,96

هموم   38 هموم النفس 38

هواء   هواء الحمّام 122-123 هواء فاسد 412 ← برد، حمّام، طبيعة، مزاج

هاج: هيّج ←   حرارة

هائج   391

وجع ←   طحال

وجوه   الوجوه المقبولة 169-170 ← حمر، حمرة، قل، هبجّ

دعة   748

أوردة ←   خارجة، داخل

أوراد ←   خارجة، داخل، عفونة

ورشكين   507,597

ورم: تورّم   تورّم الصدغين 503

ورم   42,185,186,386 ورم الأرنبة 184

أورام ←   حمّى

وصل: اتّصل   44,71

اتّصال لاتّصال الشريانات بالقلب 44-45

أوعية الأوعية المجاورة للقلب 352

وقت 251,254,324,529,645 والوقت من السنة 183
وقت الحمّى 245 وقت الغذاء 250 وقت
انحطاط نوبة الحمّى 250 وقت انكسار الحمّى
275 وقت سورة المرض 276,295 وقت
المجاهدة بين الطبيعة والمرض 297 وقت النوبة
405,770 وقت السورة 431

أوقات 262 أوقات الفترات بين نوائب الحمّى 247-248
أوقات نوبة الحمّى 248 أوقات فترات 249
أوقات طيّبة من النهار باردة رطبة 253

ولد: تولّد 15,22,193,199,205,206,337,356,366,370,476,
485,489,498,600,620,626,627,632,660,681,721
,722, 726-727, 729, 745, 756, 762, 764, 766
ولّد 193,200,201,360,732, 734,768 → حمّى،
طبيعة

وَلَد → طبيعة

وهج 586 وهج الشمس 51 وهج السموم 54 →
مطبوخات

وهن وهنا شديدا 78

وهى: أوهى 621

ييس 171,174 فإن غلب اليبس على أدمغتهم 446

يبس: يبّس　　　الأشياء الميبّسة 181

يابس　　　357,361,559,611,615 ← طبيعة، عفونة

أيد ←　　　رياحين

يدان　　　تنزل اليدان والرجلان في ماء 558 ← أطراف

يرقان　　　332,462

ينبوع:　　　ينبوع الحيات 24 ينبوع الحسّ والحركة 25-26

ينبوع القوّى الطبيعية الأربع 26-27

يوم　　　يوم النوبة 398,419,707

أيام　　　أيام الترك 413 أيام النوائب 428,694

INDEX OF PROPER NAMES

جالينوس 11, 229,256, 480

كتابه في فصول الحمّيات 480

كتابه في البحران 229

GLOSSARY OF TECHNICAL TERMS

abatement (of the fever) 117,133

absinth 128,137,138 (- decoction) 137 (-pastilles) 137

abundance → blood

acorns → suppositories

activities (natural - of the body) 7,97 (of the organs) 8

aetiology 5,6,19 → ephemeral fever

affliction 120

afflictions 19,21,22,115 (psychical) 98 (worry, grief, insomnia) 101

age 18,20,21,106,117,122,133 (young) 129 (advanced) 129

agrimony (- pastilles) 129,137

air (hot) 11 (of the bathhouse) 103 (cold) 103 (mild) 109 (corrupt) 117 → bathhouse

almond 119

aloe (- infusion) 137 (- electuary) 137 (- pastilles) 137

alum 10,98

amphemerinos → quotidian fever

amusement (providing joy and comfort) 105

aneth 103,112,129,132,135-138

anger 10,101,105 (great) 98

anise (pastilles of -) 129,136 → electuary

anointing 104 (of the heads) 103

anxiety 15

appetite 13

apples 120

ardent fever 11-13,106-114 (authentic and false) 12,107 (bilious, mucous) 12 (treatment of -) 12 (two kinds of -, authentic and severe, false and light) 12,107 (very dangerous and frightening) 13,107 (high and severe) 13,110 (symptoms of -) 107 (solid and continuous) 107 (similarity and difference between - and continuous tertian fever) 114

aridness 105

Armenian earth 110

armpit → fever

arteries 7,99 → black bile, blood, fevers, putrefaction, veins

asthma 18 (mostly caused by the heat of the chest, heart and lungs) 121-122 autumn 16,116,127

bandages (on the legs) 112,125
barberry (pastilles of -) 136
barley 110 (- broth) 106,110,130,131,135,137 (broth of fortified -)
    108, 117, 124 (gruel of parched -) 111, 113 (- dough) 111
    (- extract) 112 (meal of -) 104,112,113,125,126 (husked -)
    118,124,125
basilic vein → bleeding
bath 10,101,102-105 (with sweet waters) 103 (sweet water -)
    105
bathhouse 102,103 (with moderately heated air and water) 105
    (with moderate [hot] air) 105 → air, heat
bathing (in waters which obstruct the pores of the skin) 9,10,98
    (in waters mixed with hot ingredients) 10 (of the body, feet)
    11 (in astringent drying waters) 100
beet 112,118 (oblong pieces of -) 132
bile 116 (disturbances in -) 12
bindweed 132,135
birds (meat of -) 132
black bile 9,128,129 (superfluous) 19 (evacuation of the
    superfluous -) 20 (putrefied - within the veins and arteries,
    and outside) 127 → clysters, matter, putrefaction
bleeding 18,20,122 (of the basilic vein or the median cubital
    vein) 131
blockage → pores
blood 7,9,99,100,116,121,132,128 (role and importance of the -
    for the body) 16 (substance with which the body feeds itself)
    16,120 (best balanced element, sweetest in taste) 16,120
    (intrinsically well-tempered) 17,120 (abundance of -) 17
    (putrefied) 17,18,121 (boiling of the -) 18 (extraction of the
    superfluous -) 18 (- increases in quantity and its quality is
    modified) 121 (unripe and undigested) 121 (is by nature inside
    the veins and arteries) 121 (pure) 121 (extraction of -)
    122,123,131 (not sharp) 124 (disease of the -) 130 (burning
    of the -) 131 (coarse burned) 131 (the pure and watery part
    of the -) 134 → decoctions, fever, putrefaction, urine
blood fever 16-18,20,120-127 (treatment of -) 18 (symptoms
    preceding - and following its occurrence) 122 → drinks, pills,
    synochous fever
body   7,98,99,100,101,109,120,121,126,129,133,134,136
    (external and internal parts of the -) 7,97 (lean) 15,115 (of a

bilious nature) 15 (heaviness and fullness of the -) 18 (empty and clean) 118 (lean, dry and firm) 127 → activities, blood, exertion, fever, health, pores, pouring, veins

bodies 99,101,103,128 (outside of the -) 98,99 (thin, arid and dry) 110 (thin) 101 → massage, pouring, rubbing

borax 118

bout 19,21,115,117,118,131-133,135-138

bouts 15,116-118,128,127,131 → intervals

bowels 123 (relaxation of the -) 12,136 (rumbling in the -) 135,136 → drugs,

brain 99,126 → dryness

bramble 112

bran 112,116,118

bread (- pulp) 102,108,117,119 (washed - pulp) 110 (- crumbs) 111,112,124,126

burning fever 14,114

camomile 102,103,125,129-131,135,137

camphor 104,106,126,137 (- pastilles) 104,136

cardia (of the stomach) → stomach, veins

cataplasms 125

catarrh 103

catarrhs → chest

causes (physical and psychic) 10 (psychic) 11

cedrat (- pulp) 113

celery 128,131,136 (peels of - roots) 137

chest (free of catarrhs and cough) 125 → asthma, disease

chickens 143 (meat of -) 103,105,106

chickpeas 132

childbirth 9

clothes (covering with -) 103

clyster 10,112,118,119 (a strong - that brings the matter down) 132 (soft) 135

clysters 16,18,20,124 (that purge the black bile) 129 (relieving) 130

coalfires 103

cold 14,99,102,103,114,128,131,133,134,136,137 (severe) 9,19, 98,127,134 → morning, temperament

comfort 21,134

complexion 99 (red) 101 (pale) 101,128 (ugly) 101 (grey as lead) 134

constipation 13,20 → nature

consumption (continuous - of hot food) 10,98-99
contraria contrariis curantur 5,11
cooking 129,130 → matter
coriander (fresh) 119
costus 132
cough 119 (dry) 13,114 → chest
country 106 (hot) 129 → nature, temperament
countries (hot and dry) 15 (cold) 129
crisis 13 → disease, times
crystalline sugar 102,104,106,111,113,117,119,129,125,127
    (pulverised -) 110
cubeb pepper 137
cucumber 113,118,119,129,125 (kernels of -) 102 (pith of - seed)
    126
cumin → electuary
cupping (instead of venesection) 123

dates (green) 126
death → fever
decoction 116,130 (- of roots) 128,129,137 (to relieve nature)
    116 (which purges the burned yellow bile without harshness)
    130 (soft reliable) 136 → absinth
decoctions 16,22 (which make the blood thin and remove its
    sharpness and temper its blazing heat) 131
diagnosis 6,20
diarrhoea 15,119,120 (with the colour of gall) 116
diet 11,16 (three criteria for determining the -) 108
digestion 129
disease 9,10,11,12,17,18,98,99,106,108,117,118,120,123,132
    (treatment of the -) 6 (degree of strength...to fight the disease,
    duration of the disease, quality of the disease) 13,108,109
    (crisis of the -) 13,109 (four phases of a -) 13,107 ([acute])
    110 (paroxysm of the -) 111,112,118,122 (the beginning of
    the -) 116,117,123,129,135,137 (climax of the -) 123 (in the
    chest) 124 (duration of the -) 129 (end of the -) 130 (phlegmatic)
    131 (protracted) 138 → blood, fever
diseases 5,17,98 (all the diseases *a capite ad calcem*) 1 (sexual)
    1 (treatment of the -) 6 (sharp) 12 (in the internal organs) 97
    (external) 97 (acute) 108 → treatment
drink 104,108,110-112,117-120,123,128,129,136-138 (cold) 127
drinks 117,129 (cooling) 16,18,20 (hot) 20,100 (- which heat the
    blood) 99 (medicinal) 102 (of a balanced temperament) 106

→ foods

drug (cooling and softening) 124

drugs 22,126,129 (cold astringent) 120 (which open the obstruction, make the urine stream, and strengthen the bowels) 132 (- that are especially good for purifying the liver, softening the matter and expelling the urine) 136 (- that are good for someone whose stomach is upset) 138

dryness 105 (prevailing over his brain) 119

duck-weed 104,112,113

dyscrasia → fever

eating (abstain from -) 132 → fasting

Egyptian willow 102,113

electuary 127 (prepared with cumin) 129 (cumin-electuary) 132 (prepared with the three peppers) 132 (anise-electuary) 132 → aloe

electuaries 132

element → blood, nature (hot bilious) 115

emetics 22

emotions (excessive) 10,98,105

endive 104,128,130,131,136

ephemeral fever 8-10,97-106 (milk-fever) 9 (two kinds of -) 9,98 (three possible causes of -) 9-10,98,99 (aetiology of -) 10 (due simply to overheating of the body) 10 (symptoms of -) 10,99,106 (different causes of -) 10 (treatment of the different kinds of -) 11 (treatment of -) 99,106

ephemeral fevers 17

errhine 112

errhines 11

erysipelas 122,127

evacuation 108 → black bile

evaporations (hot, natural) 100

exercise (moderate physical) 104

exertion 10,98,115 (of body or mind) 10 (bodily) 100 (physical) 104

extraction → blood

eyelids (dry) 101

eyes (feel hot) 11 (bulging, quickly moving) 101 (hollow and motionless) 101 (dry) 101 (hollow) 101 (bulging) 122 → phantasms

face (dry, hot) 11

faces 101 (red) 99 (pleasant) 105 (swollen) 134
faculty (attractive, retentive, digesting, excretory) 98
faculties (psychical) 7,97 (four natural) 98
fainting 13,114,120
fārūq-theriac → theriac
fasting 131 → eating
fatigue 115
fear 101
feet 103,112,119,125,131,134,135,137 → massage, rubbing
fennel 130,131,136 (peels of - roots) 137
fever 16,20,97,109,116,133 (discussion of -) 7,8 (the most dangerous disease, the messenger of death...) 7,97 (a strange heat...) 7 (a disease arising from a hot dyscrasia...an unnatural heat arising from the heart) 7 (unnatural heat affecting the body) 7 (harmful for the natural activities) 7 (putrefactive) 8 (hectic) 8 (original and accidental -) 8 (humoral) 8 (nature, times of the -) 13 (hot) 121 (intermittent) 21,121,133 (following inflammations of the groin, armpit, neck) 99 (difference between - originating from boiling of the blood and that originating from putrefaction) 122 → abatement, ardent fever, blood fever, burning fever, ephemeral fever, intervals, quartan fever, quotidian fever, tertian fever
fevers 1,6,8,9,19,20,98 (mixed) 6 (three-fold division of -) 8 (two-fold division of -) 9 (putrefying - within the arteries and veins) 17 (putrefying) 17,22 (humoral) 21 (two kinds of putrefying -) 121 → regimen, treatment
fish (freshwater -) 105
flatulence 135,136
fleawort (- leaves) 102,119 (mucilage of - seed) 104,110,112, 113,118, 119, 123,125,126 (- seed) 104,110,117,119
fluid (sickening) 16
food 13,100,104,110,112,113,117,118,123,138 (little, hot and dry) 15 (too much) 19 (that is digested quickly) 108 (quality of the -) 109 (extremely fine) 109 (much) 109 (the need for -) 109 (large amount of -) 123 (light) 131 (some) 132 → consumption
foods 105 (heat-producing foods or drinks) 10 (hot) 100,104
foodstuff(s) (fine) 18,131 (fine, quickly digested and of good substance) 124
foot-baths 16
forehead 112,119,125,126 → rubbing
francolin(s) 132 (meat of -) 102,106

frost (severe) 100,103,134
fury 101,105

gall → diarrhoea
gallnuts 100
gillyflower 103
goats ([the meat of] -) 105,106
gourd 102,104,106,111,113,117-119,126 (- peels) 104, 112,113,
125 (- seed) 119 (roasted) 124,127 (pith of - seed) 126
grapes 118,124 (unripe, sour -) 103,113,120 (winter -) 110, 119,
130
grief 101,105 → afflictions
groin → fever, inflammation
gruel → barley
gum Arabic 126
gum tragacanth (white) 127

habit 106,122
hand 100 (heat of the -) 108
hands 125,134
head 119,125 (burning) 11 (heavy) 122
heads (warm) 99 (containing phlegm) 102 → anointing, heaviness,
pouring
headache 12,18,99,102,112,119,122,125
health (of the body) 13
heart 7,99,100,131 → asthma, vessels
heat 16,18,22,99,100,133,134 (in the summer) 9 (of the sun)
10,98,99,102,102 (of the bathhouse) 10 (loss of -) 10
(continuous) 12,106,107 (intense blazing) 14,116 (asthmatic)
18,121 (excessive) 98 (innate) 98 (burning - of a hot sandstorm)
99 (intense) 101 (of the stomach) 110,112,120 (strong) 117
(of the surface of the body) 122 (blazing) 136 → fever, oils
heaviness 19 (in the heads) 99-100 → body, members
honey 137 (prepared with spices) 128 (boiled with spices) 138
→ oxymel, roses, violet(s)
horse-fennel 128
humour 128 (superfluous) 103 (bilious) 107,114 (hot yellow)
114 (bilious sharp) 115
humours 8,9,17,100,116 (burning of the -) 128,132 → putrefaction

Indian laburnum (core of reedy -) 108 (core of purified -) 111,116,
118,124,130

indolence 18,122
inflammation 8,18,99,114,115,119,122,125 (of the groin) 106
inflammations → fever
infusion 100,111,137
infusions 117
ingredient 120
ingredients 110,111 (- that have a strengthening effect and that
    remove the superfluities) 138
insomnia 12,13,15,112,129 → afflictions
intercourse (sexual) 105
intervals (in the - between the bouts of fever) 109

jasmine 103
jaundice 13,114,120
joints → pain
joy → amusement
juice 102-106,108,110-113,117,118,123,125-128,130-132,135-
    137 (inspissated) 120,126
jujube 108
juveniles 107

kausos 12,114

lac (- pastilles) 129
lambs (meat of one-year-old -) 132
laxatives 20
legs 112 → bandages, rubbing
lemon-grass 129,137
lentils (husked) 113
lethargy 125
lettuce 113,119 (core of -) 102 (- seed) 113,119
licorice 126
lily 103
limbs 6 (- of the body) 6
liver 100,104,113,136 (pricking sensation in the -) 14,116
    (concave part of the -) → drugs, pneuma, veins
lung (cavity of the -) → veins
lungs 121 → asthma, veins
lycium 111,118

manna 116,130
manna from Khurāsān 108,111,118,124,135

marjoram 103,112

massage (of the bodies) 105 (of the feet) 125

mastic 138 (- pastilles) 137

matter 130,131,136,137 (putrefying) 115,118 (outside the veins) 115 (superfluous) 128,135,136 (coarse) 129 (mature) 131 (every -, whether it consists of phlegm, yellow or black bile, when it putrefies, acquires [the quality of] cooking) 133 → clyster, cooking, drugs, nature, vomiting

measles 127

meat → birds, chickens, francolins, goats, lambs

median cubital vein → bleeding

medicine 1 (ancient and Byzantine) 5 (modern) 9 (Islamic) 13,16 (methods of -) 97 (preventive) 117

melilot 130,137

members 128 (heaviness and fullness of the -) 122

milk 119 (the - of a woman who is breastfeeding a girl) 119 (of women or donkeys) 125

mint 129

moisture 99,101,103,134 → bile

morning 109,117,118 (cold of the -) 109

mouth (dry) 113,135 (sweet taste in his -) 130

mouths (moist) 134

movement 98 (excess of bodily -) 10,98

mucilage → fleawort, quince

mungo bean(s) 119,130

myrobalan (yellow) 116

myrtle 106,113,120

nard 138

natron 10,98,111,118 (pounded) 112

nature 17,120,121,122 (human) 106 (of the patient) 108,109,111, 112,117-119,123,124,135,136 (of the element that causes the fever) 115 (to relieve -) 116,131 (if the - of the patient is constipated) 117,123 (of the country) 127 (of the actual weather) 122,129,131 (if the - of the patient suffers from constipation) 111,130,132 (of the time [of the year]) 133-134 (of the phlegm) 134 (of the matter) 136 → body, decoction, fever, phlegm

nausea 135,136

neck → fever

nenuphar 102,105,112,113,119,125

nose 113,119,125,126

noses 99,102
nosebleed 12,126
nutrition 121

obstruction → drugs, pores
occupation (of the patient) 115
old man 131,133
old men → phlegm
oil 102,103,105,111-113,118,119,124,125,128,135,138
oils 119,125 (of a moderate heat) 103 (hot - which open the
    pores and attract perspiration) 132
orache 104,119,130
organ 136
organs 8,121 (of the body) 7 (main) 8 (internal) 97 (sensory)
    115,128 → diseases
overheating (of the body) 8 → ephemeral fever
oxymel 23, 130, 131 (prepared with sugar) 104, 130, 135, 136
    (- syrup prepared with honey) 128,136,137 (prepared with
    honey) 132,137

pack 112,113 (warm) 104
packs (moderately warm and fragrant) 138
pain 19,97 (constant, heavy - in the joints) 100 → spleen, stomach
palmtree (flowers) 126
palpitation 13,113,126
paroxysm → disease
pastilles 127,129,136 (tested for alleviating blood fever) 126 →
    agrimony, anise, absinth, barberry, camphor, rhabarber,
    rose(s), sandalwood, ṭabāshīr
pathology (modern) 11
patient 11,13,14,15,20,21,104,108,109,111,113,115-120,124-
    126,130,131,134-138 (condition of the -) 19 (mistake of the -)
    116 → occupation, strength, temperament
patients 100,105,117,127,134
peppers → electuary
perplexity 12
perspiration 101,128 → oils
phantasms (red - appearing before one's eyes) 122
phlegm 22,128,133 (humoral) 9 (disturbances in -) 12 (vitreous
    or acid) 21 (superfluous) 22 (burning of the -) 131 (the
    domination of the - over old men by nature and over young
    men by coincidence) 133 (putrefies and becomes hot) 134

(cold and moist) 134 (more cold and more coarse but less moist) 134 (more hot and more dry such as the salty -) 134 (salty -) 134-136 (acid) 136,137 → heads, matter, nature, putrefaction

phrenitis 13,114,116,119

physician 6,12,101,107,108,115,117,120,134 (practising) 6 (foolishness of the -) 116

physicians 5,6 (many great and excellent) 6 (Islamic) 7 (ancient and medieval) 12 (ancient) 18,121 (eminent) 133

plants (aromatic) 102 (green aromatic) 105 (cold aromatic) 119

plaster 125,126

plum(s) 102,105,108,110-112,116-120,123,124,130, 141 (black) 111

pneuma 7,8,9 (animal) 98,99 (psychical) 98 (natural) 98,100 (natural - located in the liver) 100

pneumata 7,9,97,98

pomegranate 102,112,113,117,126 (- peels) 100, 111 (seedless) 110 (sweet) 110,111,113 (bitter) 126

pomegranates (the two kinds of -) 102-106,117,118,120,123, 125,130,131

poppy 119 (- seed) 113

pores 103,104 (that which compresses the pores) 10 (obstruction of the - of the skin) 10 (open) 15,115 (blockage of the - of the body) 17 → bathing, oils

poultice (warm - around the stomach) 138

pouring (of water over the heads) 102 (of sweet lukewarm water over the bodies) 103 (of lukewarm water over his body) 130

prescriptions 14,16

pricking (sensation of -) 115 → liver, stomach

pulsation (varying - of the veins) 122

pulse 11,20 (small and fast) 11 (changes in the condition of the -) 14 (fast powerful) 18,132 (slow and very irregular) 19-20 (strong and powerful) 101 (slow) 131

pulses (weak) 101

purgations 16

purgatives 22,136

purslane 102,104,106,112,122,125,126 (- seed) 110,120,124

putrefaction 98,106,121,122 (of residues) 8 (outside the veins and arteries, and inside) 14,21,114 (of the blood within the arteries and veins) 16 (of the humours) 17 (of the blood) 18,122 (of (pure) black bile) 19,127,132 (of the (humoral) phlegm) 21,133 (of the humour(s) inside the veins and arteries,

and outside) 21,121 (of the [superfluous matter]) 127 (of
pure black, cold and dry bile) 128 (of the phlegm outside the
veins and arteries) 133 → fever

quartan fever 19-21,127-133 (natural, unnatural, extra-natural
    symptoms of -) 19,22,127 (treatment of -) 20 (continuous
    and intermittent -) 127
quince 120 (mucilage of - seed) 113,119
quotidian fever 21,22,133-138 (natural, unnatural, extra-natural
    symptoms of -) 21,133 (treatment of -) 22 (a fever which is
    called in Greek "amphemerinos", that is "the continuous")
    133 (light and delicate) 134

radish (leaves of -) 132 (sliced) 132,137
red (colour) 18,122
regimen 11,19-22,118,119,126,128,136,137 (for fevers in
    general) 13 (moist) 109 (mild) 110 (wholesome) 114 (which
    softens the stomach) 123 (very soft) 138
relaxation → bowels
rest 21,105,134
rhabarber 132 (- pastilles) 129,137
rheum (hot) 99
rose(s) 102,104,105,106,112,113,119,120,125,126,131 (- leaves)
    112,126 (preserved) 120,131,146 (preserved in honey) 128,137
    (preserved in sugar) 135 (purging - pastilles) 136 (pastilles of -)
    136
rose-water 112,113,125,126
rose-water syrup 102-105,110,113,117,119,125-127
rubbing 130 (of temples) 102 (of bodies) 103,105 (of forehead
    and temples) 112,125 (of feet and legs) 112 (of tongue) 113
    (of feet) 119 (of the body) 132 (of the soles of the feet) 135

sahj 130
salt 146 (coarsely ground) 125
sandalwood 104,106,112,120,126 (the two kinds of -) 113 (rubbed
    yellow) 126 (pastilles of -) 136
sandstorm 102 (hot) 9,98 → heat
scammony 111,118
season (of the year) 20,21,127
seasons 8
sebesten 118,124
sensation 98 (biting -) 115 → liver, stomach

senses 97

shuddering 14,114,115 (heavy) 115

skin 100,104 (dry, hot) 11 (arid and dry) 128

skins 104 (dry and arid) 100

slumber (much) 122

smallpox 122,127

sneezing (light) 131

sorrel (seed) 120

sorrow 125

soul 105 (relief to the -) 105 (healing of the -) 105

southernwood 137

spleen (pain and hardness of the -) 128

spring 16,116,130

starch 137

stomach 112,113,123,126,136,137 (pricking sensation in the -) 119 (pain in the -) 134,138 (cardia of the -) 134 (on an empty -) 135 (upset) 135,136 → drugs, heat, poultice, regimen, veins

strain 98,115

strength 13,121,136 (of the patient) 12,18,106,109,112, 116,117, 120,122 (weakness of -) 108 (degree of -) 108 (great) 116 (lack of -) 117 (healthy) 122,123 (weak) 123 (healthy and firm) 123 (weakened) 132 (confounded and weakened) 138 → disease

substance (purified) 124 (bilious) 134 → blood

sugar 118,124,132,135 (mixed with water) 104 (brown) 118 → oxymel, Sulaymān sugar, crystalline sugar

Sulaymān sugar 117,118,135 (pulverised) 110

sulphur 10,98,132

summer 15,98,107,115,129

sun 10 (burning of -) 11 (glare of the -) 99 → heat

sunburn 15

superfluity 123,126 (unripeness and crudeness of the -) 108 (fine and light) 135 (coarse and solid) 135 (mature) 137

superfluities 108,109 → ingredients

suppository 111,118

suppositories 16,18 (like acorns) 111 (soft) 124 (purging) 135

symptology 5,6,11

symptoms 12,14,15,18-22,99,101,102,115,125,128 → blood fever, ephemeral fever

synochous fever 17,18, 120-127 (continuous unbroken) 121 → blood fever

ṭabāshīr 120 (pastilles) 104,120,136 (white) 126

tamarind 108,111,116,130 (purified) 124

temperament (hot and dry) 15,115 (- and time of the year) 18 (of
the patient) 20,130 (cold - of the patient) 20,21 (of the country)
21,115,134 (natural) 106 (hot and sharp) 107 (cold and dry)
127 (of the actual weather) 127,133 (dominated by cold) 129
(dominated by yellow bile) 129 (moist and cold) 131 (cold
and moist) 133 → drinks

temples 112,119,125 (swollen) 122 → rubbing

tertian fever 14,15,20,21,114-120,129 (pure) 14,116 (intermittent)
14,114 (continuous) 14,114,115 (natural, unnatural and extra-
natural things indicating -) 15,115 (pure and impure) 15-16
(treatment of -) 16 (not pure) 116 (most dangerous and
frightening) 116 → ardent fever, things

theory (humoral) 5

theriac (known as "fārūq") 129 (*fārūq*-theriac) 132

things (warm) 116 (ripe) 128 (cooling) 129 (cooling and softening)
130 → tertian fever

thirst 12,118,120,134 (intense continuous) 106 (continuous,
unremitting) 107 (intense, continuous, and unremitting) 107
(intense) 117,129 (little) 122

throat → uvula

thyme 103,137

time (particular - of the year) 20 (- of the year) 106,117,109,122,
131 → nature, temperament

times (of the crisis [of the fever]) 13

tongue (rough) 113 (black) 113 → rubbing

tranquillity 134

transpiration 10

treatment 5,6,16,20,22,97,124,128 (- of fevers) 5 (of sharp
diseases) 12 (quality of -) 134 → ardent fever, disease, diseases,
ephemeral fever, quartan fever

tremor 14,101,114

tritaios 114

tumour 116

urine 11,20 (red fiery and fine) 14,116 (red) 18 (of those suffering
from ephemeral fever) 100 (is the wateriness of the blood)
100 (red) 101 (yellowish) 101 (stinking) 122 (red - verging
on purple) 122 (white, thin and watery) 128 (black) 128 (blond,
fire coloured) 129 (coarse and red) 130 (uncooked, coarse
and white) 131 (signs of ripeness in the -) 138 → drugs

uvula (dry - and throat) 118

vapour 101,102,103 → bile
vapours 102-104 (pure) 103 (fumy) 122
vegetables 119,137
vein → basilic, median
veins 7,107 (adjacent to the heart) 12,107,114 (of the cardia of
    the stomach) 107,115 (of the concave part of the liver) 107
    (of the cavity of the lung) 107 (inside the veins and arteries)
    114,133 (of the liver and lungs) 115 (all the - of the body)
    115 (contraction of the - faster than their expansion) 122
    (thin and concealed) 127 (full) 130 → black bile, blood, fevers,
    matter, pulsation, putrefaction
venesection 18,123 → cupping
vessels (adjacent to the heart) 115
vinegar 102,113,119,125
violet(s) 102, 104, 106, 110-113, 117-119, 124, 125, 135, 138
    (-   blossoms) 102,116,118,119,124,125,130,131,135
    (preserved) 108, 111,118,124,130,131   (- leaves) 111
    (preserved in honey) 131 → wine
vomiting 14,20,128,131,132,136-138 (constant - of bilious matter)
    116 (spontaneous) 119,135

walking (continuous) 98
washing (with astringent drying waters) 103
water 10,103,104,113,117,119,120,124-126,135,137,138 (cold)
    10, 108,110,111 (sweet [moderately] hot) 105 (lukewarm)
    105 (hot) 111,135 (warm sweet) 118,119 (warm) 131,137 →
    bath, bathhouse, pouring, sugar
waters 11 → bath, bathing, washing
water melon 106,109,112,118,125 (green and raw -) 110 (pith of
    - seed) 126
water-mint 129
way of life 21
weakness (severe) 100
weather 19,20,132 (hot and dry) 15,115 (cold and moist) 21 →
    nature, temperament
weight (loss of -) 109
wild-amaranth 106,119,130
wine (mixed with violet oil) 130 (exquisite) 138
wine vinegar 112
winter 21,129,131,133

worry 101 → afflictions
worrying (continuous) 98

year → time, temperament
yellow bile 9,17,18,116,117,128 (pure -) 12,107 (mixed with
    sweet moisture or sweet vapour) 12,107 (disturbances in -)
    12 (putrefied) 14,114 (sharp, fiery) 107 (pure in sharpness
    and pungency) 107 (because of its lightness and sharpness)
    116 (burning of -) 129-130 → decoction, matter, temperament
young man 133 (young skinny man) 129
young men 107 → phlegm

INDEX OF PROPER NAMES

'Abd al-Ġabbār 97
Abrahamow, B., 97
Abū Ja'far Aḥmad b. Abī Khālid → Ibn al-Jazzār
Alexander of Tralles 12,17
Brain, Peter 7,8,10,16
Burnett, Charles v
Conrad, Lawrence I. 4
Constantine the African v
Dietrich, Albert 3
Fleischer, H.L. 2
Freytag, G.W. 110
Galen 5,7,8,10-17,19-22,97,108,109,121
Green, Monica 5
Grmek, Mirko D. 11
Grotzfeld, H. 11
Ḥaddād, Sāmī Ibrahīm 3
Helmreich, G. 13
Hinz, Walther 110,111,124
Hippocrates 13
Ibn al-Jazzār v,5-22
Ibn Sīnā 5-16,18-21
Isḥāq ibn Sulaymān al-Isrā'īlī 2,9,17
Kühn, C.G. 5,7,8,11,13-17,19-22
Lane, E.W. 120
Langermann, Y. Tzvi 8,17
Latham, J.D-H.D. Isaacs 2,9,102,114
Levey, Martin 104
al-Mājūsī 5-16,18-22,100
Mewaldt, I. 16
Nutton, Vivian 13
Paul of Aegina 5,14,18,20,100
Puschmann, Theodor 12
Qusṭā ibn Lūqā 10
Said, Hakim Mohammad 104
Sezgin, Fuat 3
Steinschneider, Moritz 2
Suwaysī-al-Rādī 1
Ullmann, Manfred 2,16,139,148

Uri, J. 3
Vajda, G. 3
Zayn al-ʿābidīn 3

BIBLIOGRAPHY

Abrahamow, B., "The appointed time of death (*aǧal*) according to 'Abd al-Ǧabbār. Annotated translation of *al-Muǧnī*, vol. XI, pp. 3-26," Israel Oriental Studies XIII (1993), pp. 7-37.

Alexander of Tralles: *Alexander von Tralles, Original-Text und Übersetzung nebst einer einleitenden Abhandlung*. Ein Beitrag zur Geschichte der Medizin. Von Theodor Puschmann, 2 vols., Vienna 1878-1879.

de Biberstein Kazimirski, A., *Dictionnaire Arabe-Français contenant toutes les racines de la langue arabe*. New edition, 2 vols., Paris 1960.

al-Bīrūnī, *K. al-Ṣaydana fī al-ṭibb. Al Biruni's Book on Pharmacy*. Edited with an English translation by Hakim Mohammed Said, 2 vols., Karachi 1973.

Bos, G., *Qusṭā ibn Lūqā's Medical Regime for the Pilgrims to Mecca. The* Risāla fī tadbīr safar al-ḥajj, Leiden 1992.

Idem, "Ibn al-Jazzār on women's diseases and their treatment," *Medical History*, 37,3, 1993: 296-312.

Idem, *Ibn al-Jazzār on Sexual Diseases and their Treatment*. A critical edition, English translation and introduction of Book 6 of *Zād al-musāfir wa-qūt al-ḥādir* (Provisions for the Traveller and the Nourishment for the Sedentary), London 1997.

Brain, Peter, *Galen on bloodletting. A study of the origins, development and validity of his opinions, with a translation of the three works*, Cambridge 1986.

Dietrich, A., *Medicinalia Arabica. Studien über arabische medizinische Handschriften in türkischen und syrischen Bibliotheken* (Abhandlungen der Akademie der Wissenschaften in Göttingen, Philologisch-Historische Klasse, Dritte Folge, Nr. 66), Göttingen 1966.

Idem, *Dioscurides Triumphans.* Ein anonymer arabischer Kommentar (Ende 12. Jahr. n. Chr.) zur Materia medica. Arabischer Text nebst kommentierter deutscher Übersetzung hrsg. (Abh. der Akad. der Wiss. in Göttingen, Phil. Hist. Klasse, Dritte Folge, Nr. 172). I-II, Göttingen 1988.

Dozy, R.P.A., *Supplément aux Dictionnaires arabes.* Deuxième édition. I-II, Leiden 1927.

Dugat, G., "Études sur le traité de médecine d'Abou Djafar Ah'mad, intitulé: Zad al-moçafir. La provision du voyageur," *Journal Asiatique* 5 (1853): 289-353.

Fleischer, H.L., *Catalogus codicum manuscriptorum orientalium in Bibliothecae Regiae Dresdensis*, Leipzig 1831.

Freytag, G.W., *Lexicon Arabico-Latinum I-IV*, Halis Saxonum 1830-1837.

Galen, Kühn: Kühn, C.G., *Claudii Galeni Opera Omnia*, 20 vols., Leipzig 1821-1833, repr. Hildesheim 1967.

Galen, *Galeni in Hippocratis de victu acutorum commentaria quattuor*, ed. G. Helmreich (Corpus Medicorum Graecorum V9,1), Leipzig-Berlin 1914.

Galen, *Galeni in Hippocratis de natura hominis commentaria tria*, ed. I. Mewaldt (Corpus Medicorum Graecorum V9,1), Leipzig-Berlin 1914.

Galen, *Über die medizinischen Namen*: Meyerhof, M., and J.

Schacht, "Galen über die medizinischen Namen," Arabisch und deutsch herausgegeben, *Abhandlungen der Preussischen Akademie der Wissenschaften*, nr. 3 (1931), pp. 1-43 and 1-21 (Arabic).

Green, Monica H., *The transmission of ancient theories of female physiology and disease through the early Middle Ages* (Ph.D.), Princeton University 1985.

Grmek, Mirko D., *Diseases in the ancient Greek world.* Translated by Mireille Muellner and Leonard Muellner, Baltimore and London 1989.

Grotzfeld, H., *Das Bad im Arabisch-Islamischen Mittelalter. Eine kulturgeschichtliche Studie*, Wiesbaden 1970.

Hinz, Walther, *Islamische Masse und Gewichte umgerechnet ins metrische System* (Handbuch der Orientalistik I, Ergänzungs-band I, 1). Photomechanischer Nachdruck mit Zusätzen und Berichtigungen, Leiden/Köln 1970.

Hippocrates, Littré: Hippocrates, *Oeuvres complètes d'Hippo-crate.* Traduction nouvelle avec le texte grec en regard...par É. Littré, 10 vols, Paris 1839-1861, repr. Amsterdam 1973-1989.

Ibn Sīnā, *K. al-Qānūn fī l-ṭibb*, 5 books in 3 vols., repr. Beirut n.d.

Lane, E.W., *Arabic-English Lexicon*, I, 1-8, London 1863-1879.

Langermann, Y. Tzvi, "Maimonides on the synochous fever," *Israel Oriental Studies* XIII (1993), pp. 175-198.

Latham, J.D. - H.D. Isaacs, *K. al-ḥummāyāt li-Isḥāq ibn Sulaymān al-Isrā'īlī.* Edited and translated with introduction and notes, Cambridge 1981.

Levey, M., *The medical formulary or* Aqrābādhīn *of al-Kindī*. Translated with a study of its materia medica, Madison, Milwaukee and London 1966.

Al-Mājūsī, *Kāmil al-ṣinā'a al-ṭibbīya*, repr. from MS A.Y. 6375 Istanbul University Library (Publ. of the Inst. for the Hist. of Arab. Isl. Science, ed. by F. Sezgin, Series C: Facs. Editions, Vol. 16, 1-3), Frankfurt am Main 1985.

Paul of Aegina, *De re medica*: Paulus Aegineta, *De re medica* ed. I.L. Heiberg, I-II (Corpus Medicorum Graecorum IX), Leipzig-Berlin 1921-1924.

Said, *al-Biruni's Book on Pharmacy*: see al-Bīrūnī, *K. al-Ṣaydana fī al-ṭibb*.

Sezgin, Fuat, *Geschichte des arabischen Schrifttums*, Band III: *Medizin - Pharmazie - Zoologie - Tierheilkunde bis ca. 430 H.*, Leiden 1970.

Steinschneider, Moritz, *Die hebräischen Handschriften in Berlin*, Berlin 1878.

Idem, "Schriften der Araber in hebräischen Handschriften, ein Beitrag zur arabischen Bibliographie," *ZDMG* 47 (1893): 335-384.

Suwaysī - al-Rāḍī (eds.), Zād al-musāfir wa-qūt al-ḥāḍir (bks. 1-3), Tunis, *al-dār al-'arabīya li-l-kitāba*, 1986.

Ullmann, Manfred, *Die Medizin im Islam* (Handbuch der Orientalistik I, Ergänzungsband VI, 1), Leiden/Köln 1970.

Idem, *Islamic medicine*, Edinburgh 1978.

Uri, J., *Bibliothecae Bodleianae codicum orientalium, videlicet Hebraicorum, Chaldaicorum, Syriacorum, Aethiopicorum, Arabicorum, Turcicorum, Copticorumque catalogus*, vol. 1,

Oxford 1787.

Vajda, G., *Index général des manuscrits arabes musulmans de la Bibliothèque Nationale de Paris,* Paris 1953.